Principles and Practices of
Premalignant and Malignant Disorders of Vulva

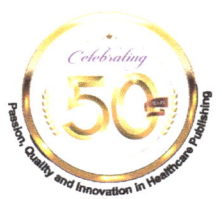

Principles and Practices of Premalignant and Malignant Disorders of Vulva

Sabera Khatun
MBBS FCPS (Obs & Gynae)
Fellow (Gynecologic Oncology)
Chairman, Department of Gynecological Oncology
Bangabandhu Sheikh Mujib Medical University,
Central Hospital
Dhaka, Bangladesh

Chief Editor
Jonathan S Berek
MD MMS
Laurie Kraus Lacob Professor
Director, Stanford Women's Cancer Center
Director, Communication and Special Programs
Stanford Comprehensive Cancer Institute
Chair, Department of Obstetrics and Gynecology
Stanford University School of Medicine
Stanford, California, USA

Co-Editors

Noor-E-Ferdous
Assistant Professor
Department of Obstetrics and Gynecology
Bangabandhu Sheikh Mujib Medical University
Dhaka, Bangladesh

Farhana Khatun
Assistant Professor
Department of Obstetrics and Gynecology
Bangabandhu Sheikh Mujib Medical University
Dhaka, Bangladesh

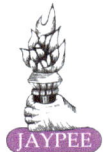

JAYPEE BROTHERS MEDICAL PUBLISHERS
The Health Sciences Publisher
New Delhi | London | Panama

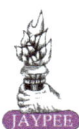

Jaypee Brothers Medical Publishers (P) Ltd

Headquarters
Jaypee Brothers Medical Publishers (P) Ltd
4838/24, Ansari Road, Daryaganj
New Delhi 110 002, India
Phone: +91-11-43574357
Fax: +91-11-43574314
Email: jaypee@jaypeebrothers.com

Overseas Offices

J.P. Medical Ltd
83 Victoria Street, London
SW1H 0HW (UK)
Phone: +44 20 3170 8910
Fax: +44 (0)20 3008 6180
Email: info@jpmedpub.com

Jaypee-Highlights Medical Publishers Inc
City of Knowledge, Bld. 235, 2nd Floor
Clayton, Panama City, Panama
Phone: +1 507-301-0496
Fax: +1 507-301-0499
Email: cservice@jphmedical.com

Jaypee Brothers Medical Publishers (P) Ltd
Bhotahity, Kathmandu, Nepal
Phone: +977-9741283608
Email: kathmandu@jaypeebrothers.com

Website: www.jaypeebrothers.com
Website: www.jaypeedigital.com

© 2019, Jaypee Brothers Medical Publishers

The views and opinions expressed in this book are solely those of the original contributor(s)/author(s) and do not necessarily represent those of editor(s) of the book.

All rights reserved. No part of this publication may be reproduced, stored or transmitted in any form or by any means, electronic, mechanical, photocopying, recording or otherwise, without the prior permission in writing of the publishers.

All brand names and product names used in this book are trade names, service marks, trademarks or registered trademarks of their respective owners. The publisher is not associated with any product or vendor mentioned in this book.

Medical knowledge and practice change constantly. This book is designed to provide accurate, authoritative information about the subject matter in question. However, readers are advised to check the most current information available on procedures included and check information from the manufacturer of each product to be administered, to verify the recommended dose, formula, method and duration of administration, adverse effects and contraindications. It is the responsibility of the practitioner to take all appropriate safety precautions. Neither the publisher nor the author(s)/editor(s) assume any liability for any injury and/or damage to persons or property arising from or related to use of material in this book.

This book is sold on the understanding that the publisher is not engaged in providing professional medical services. If such advice or services are required, the services of a competent medical professional should be sought.

Every effort has been made where necessary to contact holders of copyright to obtain permission to reproduce copyright material. If any have been inadvertently overlooked, the publisher will be pleased to make the necessary arrangements at the first opportunity. The **CD/DVD-ROM** (if any) provided in the sealed envelope with this book is complimentary and free of cost. **Not meant for sale.**

Inquiries for bulk sales may be solicited at: jaypee@jaypeebrothers.com

Principles and Practices of Premalignant and Malignant Disorders of Vulva

First Edition: **2019**

ISBN: 978-93-5270-613-6

Dedicated to

My parents Mr Sohrab Ali Sarker and Begum Nargis Ashar, who sacrificed their whole life towards making my life successful. Next to Allah, I remember them. They taught me to stand up for what is right, inspired me to do something new and good and taught me the value of time, honesty and sincerity.

Foreword

Vulva is an exposed part of the female genital tract. It has similarity with skin of the other parts of the body. Skin of vulva is a specialized structure and it is exposed to various types of external trauma and chemicals. As it is a part of skin, it is susceptible to similar types of skin diseases, Vulvar diseases are dealt with by the general gynecologists and venereologists. But most of the premalignant and malignant conditions are dealt with gynecological oncologists. Vulvar diseases are mostly neglected among all gynecological diseases.

Most of the premalignant conditions are not life-threatening but gives tremendous sufferings to the patients. Moreover these diseases are not well understood, not well studied, as well as risk factors and causes are not well established. Most of the premalignant conditions are not curable due to absence of specific treatment for the conditions. Malignant conditions of vulva, though curable in its early stage, women do not come in that stage. When they come the condition is not often curable. Even if they come in early stage; many physicians are not aware of the disease and do not advice proper and timely investigations, thus making delay in diagnosis.

Prof. Sabera Khatun has taken a bold step in writing a book on vulvar diseases. I hope that this book written by Prof. Sabera khatun on *Principles and Practices of Premalignant and Malignant Disorders of Vulva* will meet the demand of practicing gynecologists and gynecological oncologists.

This book can also be helpful to the postgraduate students of general obstetrics and gynecology, gynecological oncology and dermatology, and would be well accepted in medical circle.

TA Chowdhury
FRCS FRCOG FRCP FCPS (B) FCPS (P)
Senior Consultant (Honorary)
Department of Obstetrics and Gynecology
BIRDEM Hospital
Dhaka, Bangladesh

Preface

Diseases of the vulva in gynecologic oncology is a neglected chapter. I love gynecologic oncology, a lovely subject, becoming more and more acceptable since its first establishment. Management of gynecological cancer patients needs a multidisciplinary team to provide proper diagnosis, treatment, postoperative care, including adjuvant treatment and lastly, proper follow-up. Till now, the common gynecological cancers are addressed in different trainings, seminars, symposiums, and conferences. As vulvar cancers are only 1–2% of gynecological cancers, research works are also very scanty on this issue. My intention was to provide a comprehensive and practical book to guide the students, trainees and ultimately practitioners and gynecologic oncology workers about premalignant and malignant conditions of the vulva. With this purpose, this handbook on *Principles and Practices of Premalignant and Malignant Disorders of Vulva* was written.

As the main contributor, I tried to include all the cancers of the vulva, as well as all the surgical and medical aspects of vulvar disease. Another major contributor of this book, Professor Jonathan S Berek is the writer of Gynecologic Oncology textbook. I took much help from this book and tried to make the subject easier for my students.

Moreover, I tried to make a simple book about vulvar premalignant and malignant disorders, so that both undergraduate, postgraduate and subspecialty students become benefited from this book. I am also thankful to my co-editors for their tireless efforts make this book a reality.

Sabera Khatun

Acknowledgments

In connection with the writing of this handbook on *Principles and Practices of Premalignant and Malignant Disorders of Vulva*, I owe my gratitude to Jonathan S Berek, MD, MMS, Laurie Kraus Lacob Professor, Fellow, Stanford Distinguished Careers Institute, Director, Stanford Women's Cancer Center, Senior Scientific Advisor, Stanford Cancer Institute, Director, Stanford Health Care Communication Program, Stanford, California, USA, for his kind contribution to this handbook, his kind guidance, supply of references, edition, and hearty suggestion. I am highly grateful to him for his thorough check and correction of the manuscript.

I also heartily want to mention the names of my daughters Dr Sharmin Zaman Khan and Armin Zaman Khan, who have sacrificed their valuable time and allowed me to work hard to complete this book.

I am also glad and grateful to mention the name of Dr Rifat Ara for her kind cooperation in collecting the pictures for this book, which helped me immensely to complete this work. I specially thank my co-editors, without whose tireless efforts this book would never have become a reality.

I am also deeply impressed with my husband, Mr Asaduzzaman Khan for his continuous encouragement and inspiration to complete this work. I am indebted to him for his sincere help in completing this book.

I am very grateful to Shri Jitendar P Vij (Group Chairman), Mr Ankit Vij (Managing Director) and Mr Chetna Malhotra Vohra (Associate Director—Content Strategy) of Jaypee Brothers Medical Publishers, New Delhi, India, for publishing the book in limited time.

Lastly, I am thankful and pleased with Mrs Afia Akter, who showed great patience in typing, communicating with Jaypee Brothers Medical Publishers (P) Ltd., New Delhi, India, and completing this book for publication. I am also thankful to Mr Sharad for his sincere cooperation.

Contents

1. **Anatomy**   1
   - Mons Pubis *2*
   - Labia Majora *2*
   - Nerve Supply of External Genitalia *8*
   - Labia Minora *9*
   - Clitoris *11*
   - Vestibule *13*
   - Bartholin's Glands *15*
   - Female Urethra *16*

2. **Vulvar Dystrophies**   18
   - Types of Vulvar Dystrophy *18*
   - Lichen Sclerosus *19*
   - Squamous Cell Hyperplasia *27*
   - Lichen Planus *30*

3. **Non-neoplastic Inflammatory and Ulcerative Vulvar Disease**   33
   - Vulvar Vestibulitis *33*
   - Vulvar Psoriasis *34*
   - Fox–Fordyce Disease *34*
   - Crohn's Disease *34*
   - Behcet Syndrome *36*
   - Systemic Disease *38*

4. **Vulvar Intraepithelial Neoplasia**   40
   - Incidence and Etiology *40*
   - Relation between Vulvar Dystrophy, VIN and Invasive Squamous Cell Carcinoma Vulva *41*
   - Classification of Vulvar Intraepithelial Neoplasia *43*
   - Natural History of Vulvar Intraepithelial Neoplasia *44*
   - Terminology for Squamous Vulvar Intraepithelial Neoplasia *45*
   - Clinical Profile of Vulvar Squamous Intraepithelial Neoplasia *46*
   - Paget's Disease *58*

5. Vulvar Cancer (Squamous Type)   64
- Composition of Vulva   *64*
- Classification of Vulvar Cancer According to Histopathology   *64*
- Incidence and Epidemiology   *65*
- Etiology   *65*
- Diagnostic Dilemmas   *66*
- Types of Squamous Cell Carcinoma of Vulva   *67*
- Staging System   *72*
- Predicting Lymph Node Metastasis   *72*
- Treatment   *75*
- Advanced Stage Disease   *87*
- Role of Radiation Therapy in Vulvar Cancer   *94*
- Recurrent Vulvar Cancer   *98*
- Verrucous Carcinoma   *101*

6. Nonsquamous Type of Vulvar Cancer   105
- Vulvar Malignant Melanoma   *105*
- Bartholin's Gland Carcinoma   *110*
- Basal Cell Carcinoma   *112*
- Paget's Disease and Other Vulvar Adenocarcinomas   *113*
- Unusual Varieties of Vulvar Malignancy   *115*
- Metastatic Tumors of the Vulva   *116*

Index   *119*

CHAPTER 1

Anatomy

INTRODUCTION

Vulva, also known as female external genitalia include the mons pubis, the labia majora, the labia minora, the clitoris and the glandular structures that open into the vestibule of vagina. The glands, which open into the vulva are vestibular gland (Bartholins gland) and greater vestibular glands (Fig. 1.1). The size, shape and coloration of these structures vary between individuals and racial groups. External genitalia of the female have their exact counterparts in the male.

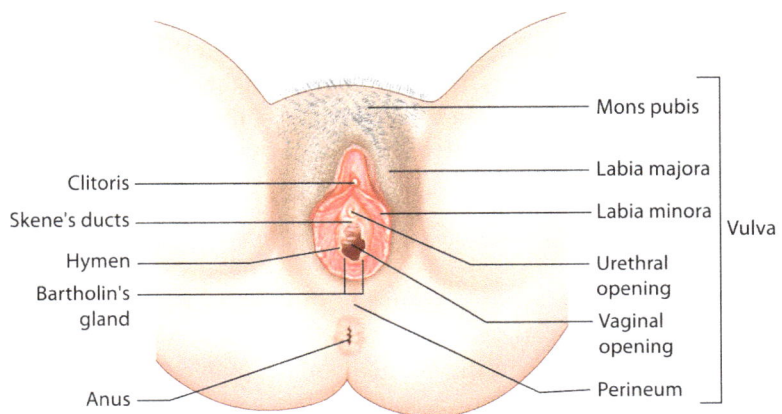

Fig. 1.1: Different parts of vulva.

The essential difference is the failure of the mid-line fusion of the genital folds in the female. The scrotum is represented by the labia majora, the corpus spongiosum by the labia minora and the bulb of the vestibule by the corresponding vessels and nerves.

The vulvar epithelium is primarily of ectodermal origin. However, the shape of the vulva is the result of condensations of subepithelial mesoderm that appear during the third and fourth weeks of embryonic life. In the development of the external genitalia, the indifferent phase, which extends from the third to the 8th week of embryonic life, begins with the development of the genital tubercle (or eminence), which is anterior to the urogenital sinus. This tubercle will become the clitoris. Both the urogenital folds (the future labia minora) and the labioscrotal folds (the future labia majora) develop between the 4th and 6th weeks of embryonic life. By the sixth week the cloacal membrane is divided into the urogenital membrane anteriorly and anal membrane posteriorly. The urethra and the vestibule (or introitus) with its mucus-secreting glands are of endodermal (urogenital sinus) origin. The structures of the vulva have all been developed by the seventh to eighth week of embryonic life. Further differentiation involves the growth of these structures.

MONS PUBIS

It is the mound of hair bearing skin and subcutaneous fat in front of the pubic symphysis and pubic bones. It contains fibro-fatty tissue with the onset of puberty. Course pubic hair grows over the mons pubis. Normal pubic hair in the female is distributed in the shape of inverted triangle with the base centered over the mons pubis. Nevertheless, in approximately 25% of normal women, hair may extend upward along the linea alba.

LABIA MAJORA

The labia majora are two rounded mound of hairy skin and subcutaneous tissue originating from the mons pubis and terminating in the perineum. It forms the boundary of the pudendum clefts and lateral boundaries of the vulva. Approximately, it is 7–9 cm long and 2–4 cm wide, varying in size with height, weight, race, age, parity and pelvic architecture. Ontogenetically these permanent folds of skin are homologous to the scrotum of the male. Both are developed from genital swelling. The lateral surfaces of the labia majora are adjacent to the medial border of the thigh, forming a deep groove when legs are together. Medial surfaces of the labia majora may oppose each other directly or may be separated by protrusion of the labia minora. The labia are joined in front as the anterior commissure, at the back they fade away behind the vagina, the connecting skin between them forming a low ridge, the posterior commissure, which extends backwards to cover the perineal body forming the region of the gynecological perineum (Fig. 1.2)

Deep Structures of Labia Majora

Inner surface of labial skin is provided with sebaceous rich follices. Underlying the skin is a thin, poorly developed muscle layer called the tunica dartas labialis, the fiber of which run at right angles to the wrinkles of the surface forming a criss-cross pattern. Deep to the dartos layer, there is a thin layer of fascia, containing large amount of adipose and areolar tissue.

Numerous sweat glands are found in the labia majora, especially on the medial aspect. In the deeper substance of the labia majora are longitudinal bands of muscle, which are continuous with the

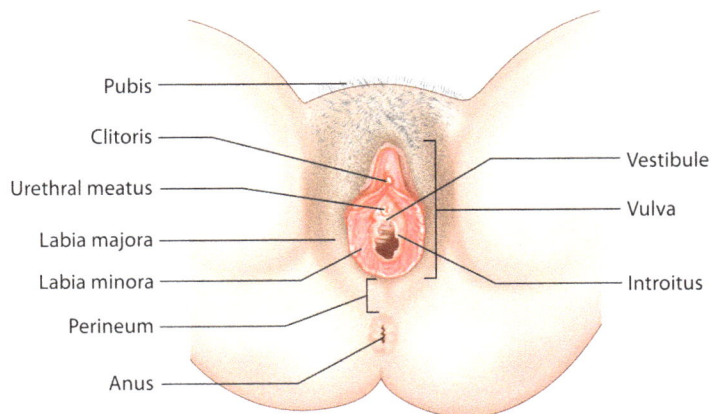

Fig. 1.2: Female external genitalia.

ligamentum teres uteri (round ligament) as it emerges from the inguinal canal.

The labia majora are longitudinal folds of fat are covered by stratified squamous epithelium, which may have varying degrees of surface maturation and keratinization and an underlying layer of connective tissue. The labia majora are virtually absent in a young child. Their development, which occurs primarily by the deposition of fat, is one of the secondary sex characteristics that herald puberty. The skin of the more prominent portions of the labia majora is pigmented and rich in hair follicles and sebaceous (holocrine) and sudoriferous glands (Figs. 1.3 and 1.4). The letter includes the unique apocrine glands, which are found only in specific areas (axilla, vulva, and perianal region). They are characterized by the presence of decapitation secretion, which means that the outer surface of the cell is shed as part of the secretory process. Because this secretion begins at puberty and because the cyclic nature of this activity follows that of the ovary, these apocrine glands may be designated accessory sex glands. An understanding of this cyclic activity is relevant to the diagnosis and treatment of certain vulvar diseases (e.g. Fog-Fordyce disease).

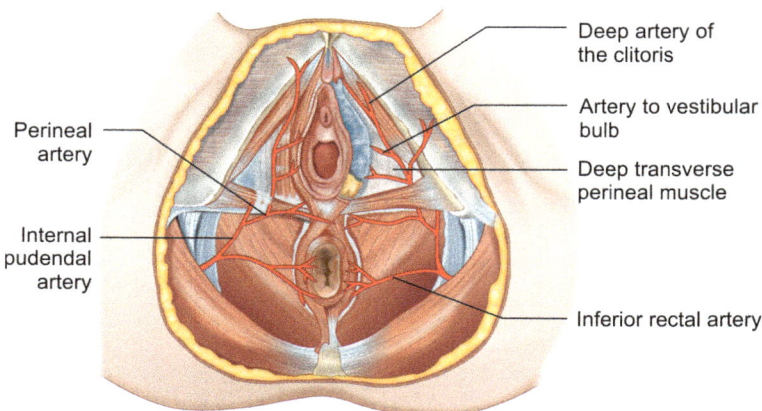

Fig. 1.3: Arteries of labia majora and vulva.

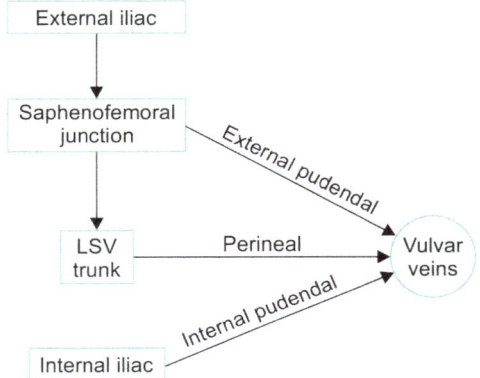

Fig. 1.4: Drainage of vulvar veins. (LSV: Long saphenous vein)

Arteries of Labia Majora

Blood supply of the labia majora comes from external and internal pudendal arteries—forming extensive anastomosis. Within the labia majora a circular arterial pattern originating inferiorly from a branch of the perineal artery, from the external pudendal artery in the anterolateral aspect and from a small artery of the ligamentum teres uteri superiorly (*see* Fig. 1.3).

Veins of Labia Majora

The venous drainage is extensive and forms a plexus with numerous anastomoses. In addition to anastomoses, the vein communicates with the dorsal vein of the clitoris, the veins of the labia minora, the perineal veins and the inferior hemorrhoidal plexus. On each side, the posterior labial veins connect with the external pudendal vein, terminating in the great sephanous vein just prior to its entrance in the fossa ovalis. This large plexus is frequently manifested by the presence of large varicosities during pregnancy (Fig. 1.4).

Lymphatics of Labia Majora

The lymphatics of the labia majora are extensive and utilize two systems, one lying superficially, under the skin and another lying deeper, within the subcutaneous tissue. From the upper two-thirds of the both-sided labia majora, superficial lymphatics pass toward the symphysis and then run laterally to join the medial superficial inguinal nodes. These nodes drain into the superficial inguinal nodes overlying the saphenous fossa. The drainage flows through the fossa ovalis to the deep subinguinal nodes of cloquet connecting with the external iliac chain. The superficial subinguinal nodes situated over the femoral trigone, also accept superficial drainage from the lower extremity and the gluteal region and may include drainage from perineum. At the symphysis pubis, the lymphatics anastomose in a plexus between the right and left nodes.

Therefore, any lesion involving the labia majora allows direct involvement of the lymphatic structures of the contralateral inguinal area. The lower part of the labium majus has superficial and deep drainage, which is shared with the perineal area. The lymphatic drainage of the perineal region passes in part, through the afferent lyphatics to the superficial subinguinal nodes. From the posteromedial aspect of the labia majus, it frequently enters the lymphatic plexus surrounding the rectum (Figs. 1.5 to 1.8).

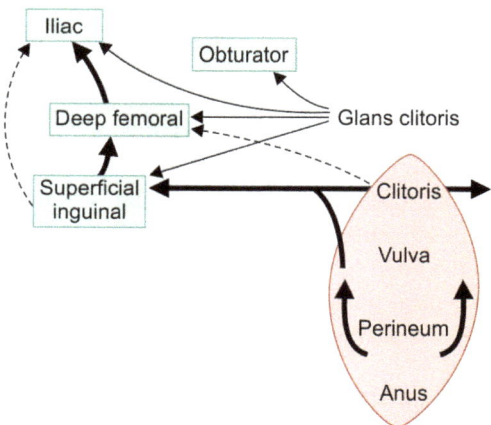

Fig. 1.5: Lymphatic drainage of clitoris.

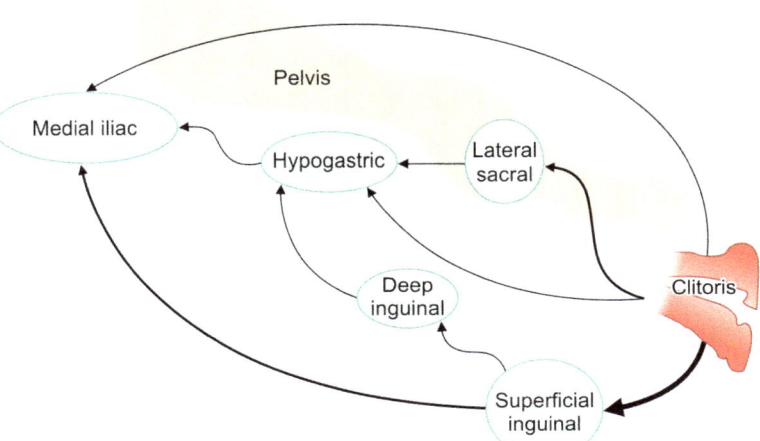

Fig. 1.6: Diagrammatic presentation of lymphatic drainage of clitoris.

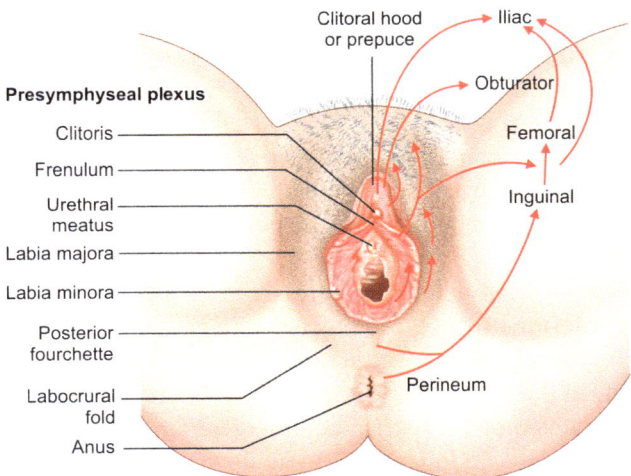

Fig. 1.7: Surface anatomy of the vulva and vulvar lymphatic flow.

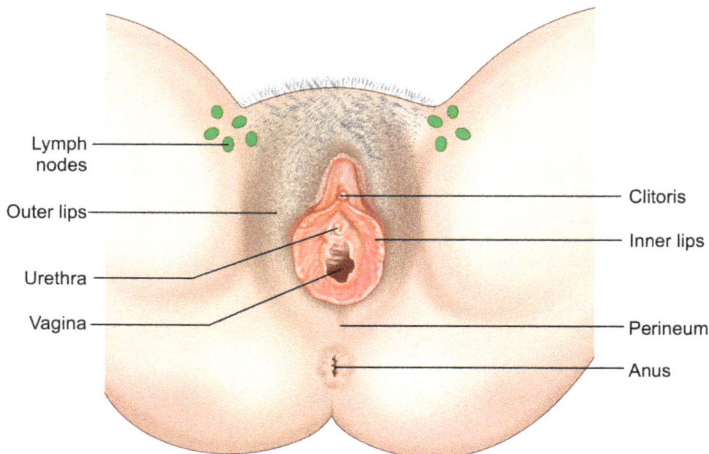

Fig. 1.8: Vulva with lymph nodes.

NERVE SUPPLY OF EXTERNAL GENITALIA

The innervations of the female external genitalia have been studied by many investigators. The iliohypogastric nerve originates from T12 and L1 and traverses laterally to the iliac crest between the transversus and internal oblique muscles, at which point it divides into two branches: the anterior hypogastric nerve, which descends anteriorly through the skin over the symphysis, supplying the superior portion of the labia majora and the mons pubis, and the posterior iliac, which passes to the gluteal area.

The ilioinguinal nerve originates from L1 and follows a course slightly inferior to the iliohypogastric nerve, with which it may frequently anastomose, branching into many small fibers that terminate in the upper medial aspect of the labium majus.

The genitofemoral nerve (L1–L2) emerges from the anterior surface of the psoas muscle to run obliquely downward over its surface, branching in the deeper substance of the labium majus to supply the dartos muscle and that vestige of the cremaster present within the labium majus. Its lumboinguinal branch continues downward onto the upper part of the thigh.

From the sacral plexus, the posterior femoral cutaneous nerve, originating from the posterior divisions of S1 and S2 and the anterior divisions of S2 and S3, divides into several rami that, in part, are called the perineal branches. They supply the medical aspect of the thigh and the labia majora. These branches of the posterior femoral cutaneous nerve are derived from the sacral plexus. The pudendal nerve, composed primarily of S2, S3, and S4 often with a fascicle of S1, sends a small number of fibers to the medial aspect of the labia majora. The pattern of nerve endings is illustrated in Table 1.1.

LABIA MINORA

Labia minora are a pair of elongated, thin and fat-free cutaneous folds situated along the medial aspects of labia majora. The cleft at the midline between two labia minora is known as vestibule, which presents the external orifices of urethra and vagina. The labia minora measure approximately 5 cm in length and 0.5–1 cm in the thickness. The width varies according to age and parity, measuring 2–3 cm at its narrowest diameter and 5–6 cm at its widest with multiple corrugations over the surface. Traced in front, each labium minus splits into upper and lower layers. The upper layer covers the upper surface of glans clitoris and meets its fellow from its opposite side to form the prepuce of clitoris; the lower layers from both sides meet and are attached to the undersurface of glans forming the frenulum of clitoris. Traced behind, the labia minora meets each other to form a fold, the frenulum of the vestibule (fourchette). During childbirth, the frenulum of the vestibule is interrupted. A deep cleft is formed at the lateral surface between the labia majus and the labia minus. The skin on the labia minora is smooth and pigmented. The color and distension vary, depending on the level of sexual excitement and the pigmentation of the individual. The glands of the labia minora are homologous to the glands of Littre of the penile portion of the male urethra.

The labia minora are composed primarily of vascular connective tissue. The surface stratified epithelium is characterized by a relative absence of the surface keratin and the underlying granular layer as well as hair follicles in the subcutaneous tissue. However, numerous sebaceous glands are present that, in the absence of hair follicles,

TABLE 1.1: Nerve supply of external genitalia.

	Touch			Pressure	Pain		Other types
	Meissner corpuscles	Market tactile disks[1]	Peri-trichous endings	Vater-Pacini corpuscles[2]	Free nerve endings	Ruffini corpuscles[2]	Dogiel and Krause corpuscles[3]
Mons pubis	++++	++++	++++	+++	+++	++++	+
Labia majora	+++	++++	++++	+++	+++	+++	+
Clitoris	+	+	0	++++	+++	+++	+++
Labia minora	+	+	0	+	+	+	+++
Hymenal ring	0	+	0	0	+++	0	0
Vagina	0	0	0	0	+ Occasionally	0	0

(*Source*: Current Obstetric and Gynaecologic Diagnosis and Treatment.)[4]

secrete their contents directly onto the skin. Apocrine glands are rare in this area.

Arteries of Labia Minora

The main source of arterial supply occurs through anastomoses from the superficial perineal artery, branching from the dorsal artery of the clitoris, and from the arteries of the medial aspect of the labia majora. Similarly, the venous pattern and plexus are extensive.

Veins of Labia Minora

The venous drainage is to the medial vessels of the perineal and vaginal veins, directly to the veins of the labia majora, to the inferior hemorrhoidals posteriorly, and to the clitoral veins superiorly.

Lymphatics

The lymphatics medially may join those of the lower third of the vagina superiorly and the labia majora laterally, passing to the superficial subinguinal nodes and to the deep subinguinal nodes. In the midline, the lymphatic drainage coincides with that of the clitoris, communicating with that of the labia majora to drain to the opposite side.

Nerve

The innervation of the labia minora originates, in part, from fibers that supply the labia majora and from branches of the pudendal nerve as it emerges from the canalis pudendalis (Alcock's canal). These branches originate from the perineal nerve. The labia minora and the vestibule area are homologous to the skin of the male urethra and penis. The short membranous portion, approximately 0.5 cm of the male urethra, is homologous to the midportion of the vestibule of the female.

CLITORIS

The clitoris is the homologous of the dorsal port of the penis and consists of two small erectile cavernous bodies, terminating in a rudimentary gland—clitorids. The erectile body, the corpus clitoridis, consists of two crura clitoridis and the glans clitoridis, with overlying skin and prepuce, a miniature homolog of the glans penis. The cura extend outward bilaterally to their position in the anterior portion of the vulva. The cavernous tissue homologous to the corpus spongiosum penis of male, appears in the vascular pattern of the labia minora in the female. At the lower border of the pubic arch, a small triangular fibrous band extends into the clitoris as suspensory ligament to separate the two crura, which run inward, downward and laterally at this point, close to the inferior rami of the pubic symphysis. The crura lie inferior to the ischiocavernosus muscles and bodies. The tip of clitoris, the glans, is highly sensitive and formed by the cephalic continuation of the bulbs of the vestibule. The glans is situated superiorly at the fused termination of the crura. It is composed of erectile tissue and contains an integument, in hood like shape termed the prepuce. On its ventral surface, there is a frenulum clitoridis, the fused junction of the labia minora.

The corpora cavernosa in both sexes are formed by enlargement of vessels in the genital tubercle (penis or clitoris). The clitoris, like its male homolog the penis, is made up of vascular erectile tissue. However, the clitoris lacks the corpus spongiosum. Nerve fibers are prominent in the clitoris, accounting for the response to tactile stimulation. The two vestibular bulbs, which are collections of veins situated beneath the anterior portion of the labial structures, are part of the corpus cavernosum.

Arteries of Clitoris

The blood supply to the clitoris is from its dorsal artery, a terminal branch of the internal pudendal artery, which is the terminal division of the posterior portion of the internal iliac (hypogastric) artery. As it enters the clitoris, it divides into two branches—the deep and dorsal arteries. Just before entering the clitoris itself, a small branch passes posteriorly to supply the area of the external urethral meatus.

Veins of Clitoris

The venous drainage of the clitoris begins in a rich plexus around the corona of the glans, running along the anterior surface to join the deep vein and continuing downward to join the pudendal plexus from the labia minora, labia majora and perineum, forming the pudendal vein.

Lymphatics of Clitoris

The lymphatic drainage of the clitoris coincides primarily with that the labia minora, the right and left sides having access to contralateral nodes in the superficial inguinal chain. In addition, its extensive network provides further access downward and posteriorly to the external urethral meatus toward the anterior portion of the vestibule.

Nerves of Clitoris

The innervations of the clitoris are through the terminal branch of the pudendal nerve, which originate from the sacral plexus as previously discussed. It lies on the lateral side of the dorsal artery and terminates in branches within the glans, corona, and prepuce. The nerve endings in the clitoris vary from a total absence within the glans a rich supply primarily located within the prepuce. A total absence of endings within the clitoris itself takes on clinical significance when the clitoris itself phases placed on the clitoris in discussing problems of sexual gratification in women.

VESTIBULE

It is an area bounded laterally by two labia minora, anteriorly by frenulum of the clitoris and urethra, posteriorly by frenulum of posterior commissure and interiorly it is bordered by the hymeneal ring. The external urethral meatus and the vaginal orifices open into the vestibule. The junction of the vagina with the vestibule is limited by membrane termed hymen. Its shape and openings vary and depend on age, parity and sexual experience. The form of the opening may be infantile, annular, semilunar, cribriform, septate or vertical. Even it may be imperforate. In parous women and in the postcoital state, the tags of the hymeneal integument are termed carunculae myrtiformes.

The external urethral orifice, which is approximately 2–3 cm posterior to the clitoris, is a slightly irregular and elevated surface with depressed areas on both sides. It may be satellite or crescentic in shape. It is characterized by many small mucosal folds surrounding its opening. Bilaterally and on the surface are the orifices of the para and periurethral glands. At approximately 5 and 7 O'clock positions, just external to the hymenal rings, are two small papular elevations that represent the orifices of the para and periurethral glands. The vaginal orifices lie behind the urethra and presents H-shaped slit. Hymen projects into the vaginal lumen close to the external orifice.

Arteries of Vestibule

The blood supply to the vestibule is an extensive capillary plexus that has anastomoses with the superficial transverse perineal artery. A branch comes directly from the pudendal anastomosis with the inferior hemorrhoidal artery in the region of fossa navicularis; the blood supply of the urethra anteriorly, a branch of the dorsal artery of the clitoris and the azygos artery of the anterior vaginal wall, also contributes.

Veins of Vestibule

Venous drainage is extensive involving the same areas described for the arterial network.

Lymphatics of Vestibule

The lymphatic drainage has a distinct pattern. The anterior portion, including that of the external urethral meatus, drains upward and outward with that of the labia minora and clitoris. The portion next to the urethral meatus may join that of the anterior urethra, which empties into the vestibular plexus to terminate in the superficial inguinal nodes, the superficial subinguinal nodes, the deep subinguinal nodes, and the external iliac chain. The lymphatics of the fossa navicularis and the hymen may join those of the posterior vaginal wall, intertwining with the intercalated lymph nodes along the rectum, which follow the inferior hemorrhoidal arteries. This pattern becomes significant with cancer. Drainage occurs through the pudendal and the hemorrhoidal chain and through the vestibular plexus onto the inguinal region.

Nerves of Vestibule

The innervation of the vestibular area is primarily from the sacral plexus through the perineal nerve. The absence of the usual modalities of touch is noteworthy. The vestibular portion of the hymenal ring contains an abundance of free nerve endings (pain).

BARTHOLIN'S GLANDS[5]

The bulbs of the vestibule are a pair of elongated erectile tissue, which embrace the sides of the vaginal orifice and are continuous in front with the glans clitoridis. The vestibular bulbs are covered superficially by bulbospongiosus muscles.

Greater vestibular glands also known as Bartholin's glands form pea-shaped masses, less than 1 cm in diameter lying at the sides of the vaginal arifice, behind the posterior end of vestibular bulb and inferior, lateral to the bulbospongiosus muscle. The gland has a duct measuring approximately 5 mm in diameter. The gland is tubular and alveolar in character, with a thin capsule. There are connective tissue septa, which divide the gland into lobules in which occasional smooth muscle fibers are found. The epithelium, lining the lobules, is cuboid or culumnar, with cytoplasm containing mucinogen droplets. The epithelium of the duct is simple cubical to stratified squamous type at its orifice.

Bartholin's glands are racemose, their lobulation is significant when surgical excision is indicated. Care must be taken to remove the entire gland. Fortunately, such surgery is rarely necessary today because incision and marsupialization of the dilated duct usually results in adequate drainage and avoids an extensive dissection. The incision for drainage should be placed in the region of the normal gland orifice at introitus, not through the skin of the labia minora. Removal is indicated only when deep-seated infections recur or when the possibility of neoplasm exists.

The stratified epithelium at the orifice of Bartholin's gland changes to transitional epithelium in the main duct. As the duct divides, the epithelium has fewer and fewer layers, and the superficial layer of cells remains columnar or cuboidal. The acini are lined by mucus-secreting epithelium, in which the nuclei are located near the basement membrane.

The secretion is a clear, viscid and stringy mucoid substance and an alkaline pH. Secretion is active during sexual activity. Nonetheless, after about age 30, the glands undergo involution and become atrophic and shrunken.

The arterial supply to the greater vestibular gland comes from a small branch of the artery on the bulbocavernosus muscle, penetrating deep into its substance. Venous drainage coincides with the drainage of the bulbocavernosus body. The lymphatics drain directly into the lymphatics of the vestibular plexus, having access to the posterior vaginal wall along the inferior hemorrhoidal channels. They also drain via the perineum into the inguinal area. Most of this minor drainage is along the pudendal vessels in the pudendal canal and explains, in part the difficulty in dealing with cancer involving the gland. The lesser vestibular glands are very small mucus glands with minute opening between the urethral and vaginal openings.

The deep perineal space is traversed by both the urethra and vagina. It contains sphincter urethrae, deep transverse perineal muscles, nerves, and vessels. The pudendal nerve and internal pudendal vessels have a distribution in the deep perineal space.

FEMALE URETHRA

The female urethra is mostly lined by transitional epithelium, but stratified squamous epithelium is present at or near the external urethral meatus. It must be appreciated that the mesoderm of the Wolffian (mesonephric) ducts contributes to the trigone and adjacent urethra and that the latter portion of epithelium responds to steroid hormone stimulation. The postmenopausal patient who has urinary tract irritation, manifested by symptoms such as urinary frequency and urgency, may achieve symptomatic relief when estrogen is used.

At each side of the border of the urethral meatus are the openings of the Skene (paraurethral) ducts, which are tiny, tortuous canals that course just beneath the urethra for a distance of about 1.5 cm. These are lined by squamous epithelium. These may be the seat of an infection that is inaccessible to treatment by local application of antibiotics. Also it has been shown that the distal urethra is almost completely surrounded by a labyrinth of minor paraurethral glands. Occlusion of one or more of these glands Skene gland cyst. Subsequent infection may result in development of a suburethral abscess that occasionally causes urinary retention in women. In cases of recurrent urinary tract infection, the paraurethral canals should be suspected as a focus of infection, especially in the absence of other pathologic lesion. This is particularly true in patients whose urinary tract infections occur after coitus. Urethral diverticula may be the locus for these infections.

REFERENCES

1. Hernandez E, Atkinson BF. Diseases of the vulva: Cornelia Trimble. In: Trimble EL, Woodruff JD (Eds). Clinical Gynecologic Pathology, 1st edition. Philadelphia: WB Saunders Company; 2009.
2. Datta AK. Essentials of Human Anatomy (Thorax and Abdomen), 8th edition. Lenin Saranee, Kolkata: Current Books International; 2011.
3. Sinnatamby CS. Last's Anatomy Regional and Applied, 10th edition. Edinburgh: Churchill Livingstone; 1999.
4. Decherney AH, Nathan L. Current Obstetric & Gynecologic Diagnosis & Treatment, 9th edition. New Delhi: McGraw-Hill Education (Asia); 2002.
5. Cohen SD, Wright F, Hernandez E, et al. Management of the Bartholin abscess. Am Gynecol Health. 1990;4:99-102.

CHAPTER 2

Vulvar Dystrophies

INTRODUCTION

The skin of the vulva is highly specialized in that it contains many different kinds of glands, nerve endings and openings of some important intra-abdominal structures. It also performs many unique functions and very sensitive and susceptible to a variety of diseases. The skin of the vulva is a site of chronic irritation and moisture that causes some chronic and resistant changes.

The term vulvar dystrophy includes a spectrum of non-neoplastic noninfective inflammatory epithelial disorders, which consist of both atrophic and hypertrophic lesions of the vulva. Usually, it is caused by a wide range of stimuli that result in circumscribed or diffuse white lesions of the vulva. Previously, the term vulvar dystrophy was used to define the non-neoplastic inflammatory epithelial disorders of the vulva.

TYPES OF VULVAR DYSTROPHY

For many years, there has been controversy in naming vulvar dystrophy and this often resulted in several terms being used to describe the same condition. In 1989, the International Society for the Study of Vulvar Diseases (ISSVD) developed new terminology to better identify these diseases and reduce patient and doctor confusion. According to ISSVD, the lesions included are:

- Lichen sclerosus (previously lichen sclerosus et atrophicus)
- Squamous cell hyperplasia (previously hyperplasic dystrophy)
- Lichen simplex chronicus
- Lichen planus
- Psoriasis.

Characteristically these patients present with intense pruritus with or without of more than one changes. Pain and characteristics skin changes like patches, plaques, reddened area or combination. Naked eye changes give little clue to the diagnosis. To differentiate different types of vulvar dystrophy and to rule out the malignant change always require histopathological confirmation. Sometimes repeated biopsy is required to conclude diagnosis and to know the result of treatment. These patients must be re-examined periodically and repeated biopsy taking is encouraged. Risk of underlying malignancy is less than 5%.

LICHEN SCLEROSUS

Lichen sclerosus is a common chronic inflammatory skin condition that most often affects vulvar and perianal skin. The disease may start at any age, although it is most often diagnosed in women over 50 years. Commonly affected women are of more than 65 years age. Prepubertal girls may also be affected, when there is history of sexual abuse.

It is 10 times more common in women than in men. 15% patients will have a known family history. It may follow or coexist other skin conditions like psoriasis, moniliasis and scabies. 20% patients are known case of other autoimmune diseases.[1]

Etiology

Exact etiology of lichen sclerosus is unknown but includes genetic, hormonal, irritant and infectious components. Most likely, it is related to autoimmune process, which has been clearly demonstrated. Autoimmune thyroid diseases are associated in 20% cases. Other autoimmune diseases like pernicious anemia or alopeciata may also be associated. Autoimmunity as an etiological role has been documented by the presence of extracellular matrix protein I (ECM-1) antibodies in 60–80% of women with vulvar lichen sclerosus.[1]

Friction or damage to the skin can bring out lichen sclerosus and make it worse. This is called a "Koebner response". It has been suggested that it may be caused by chronic intermittent damage by urine occluded under the foreskin.[2]

Pathogenesis

Commonly affected women are postmenopausal. There is decrease in endogenous estrogen, which causes atrophic change in the vulvar skin and subdermal tissues. The result is thinning of vulvar skin and contracture of vaginal introitus. Vulvar skin becomes fragile and sensitized to trauma. Therefore, scarring and trauma may elicit its development.

Clinical Features

Symptoms

Intractable soreness and pruritus are the commonest symptoms. Other symptoms are dysuria, dyspareunia and painful defecation. These are due to tear, fissure and tightening of the skin around the anus, vaginal introitus and external urethral meatus. Pruritus leads to rubbing and scratching which may lead to areas of hypertrophy and ulceration.

Sign

On examination, lichen sclerosus primarily found to involve nonhair bearing, inner areas of the vulva. It can be localized to one small area or extensively involved perineum, labia minora and clitoral hood. It can also spread on to the inner aspect of the labia majora, inguinal fold and in 50% of women to anal and perianal skin. Lichen sclerosus never involves vaginal mucosa.

During the acute phase, the lesion may appear reddish or purple in color and classically, involves non-hair bearing areas of vulva, perineum and perianal region giving rise to hour glass pattern. With chronic disease, the skin becomes thin, wrinkled and white, giving rise to cigarette-paper appearance. Vulvar structures contract with agglutination of the labia minora and prepuce causing introital stenosis (Fig. 2.1A).

Vulvar skin changes pale, thinned, atrophic, wrinkled and fragile plaques of varying sizes are developed (Fig. 2.1B).

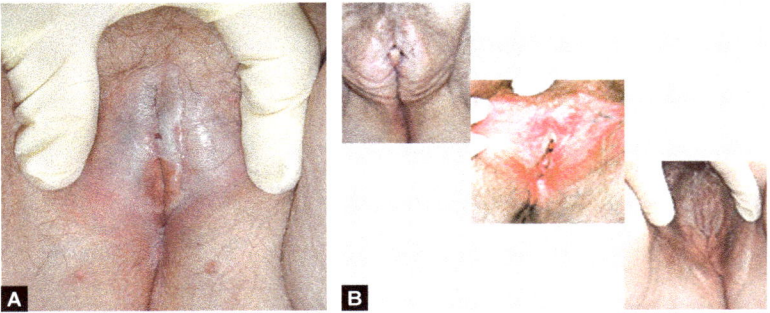

Figs. 2.1A and B: Lichen sclerosus. (A) Agglutination of the labia minora and prepuce. (B) Changes in vulvar skin and fragile plaques of varying sizes are developed.

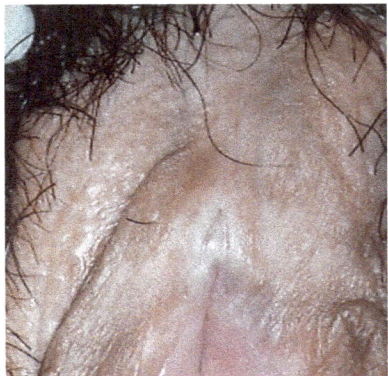

Fig. 2.2: Clitoral phimosis.

Chronic rubbing and scarring may obliterate the normal skin texture and disrupt the normal architecture. Labia minora may be fused or ultimately completely resorbed. Clitoris may be burred (Phimosis) (Fig. 2.2). Vaginal introitus become narrow and stenosed (Fig. 2.3)

Diagnosis

For definitive diagnosis, suspicious areas must be biopsied. Biopsy can be taken under local anesthesia by means of a key's punch biopsy forceps. Full thickness skin biopsy from the affected area should be taken. Usually multiple biopsy is required for confirmation of the diagnosis.

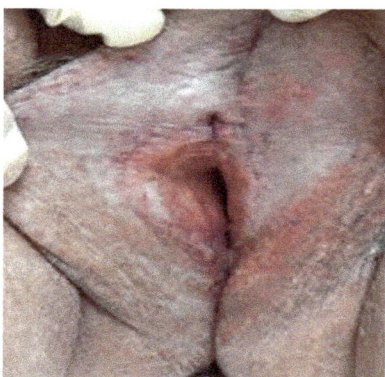

Fig. 2.3: Stenosed vaginal introitus.

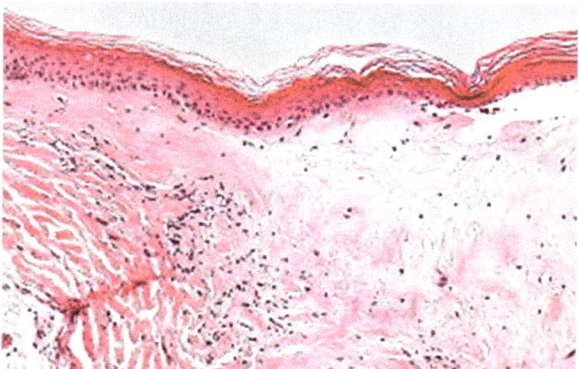

Fig. 2.4: Microscopic feature of lichen sclerosis.

Histologically, though this is primarily one of atrophy of the skin, thus areas of dysplasia may develop. So, biopsy is mandatory.

Lichen sclerosis is a histopathological diagnosis. In a well-developed lesion, classic histopathological features from superficial to deeper layers are (Fig. 2.4):
- Hyperkeratosis
- Atrophy of the superficial epithelium
- Hydropic degeneration of the basal cells
- Pale-staining homogeneous zone in the upper dermis
- Inflammatory mainly monocytic cell infiltration in the lower dermis
- Flattening of the rete pegs.

Differential Diagnosis

Differential diagnosis requires thorough evaluation of history, clinical examination findings and histological findings. Following different conditions should be considered for the diagnosis of lichen sclerosis.
- Erosive or advanced lichen planus
- Scarring cicatricial pemphigoid
- Lichen simplex
- Advanced scleroderma
- Lupus erythematosus
- Radiation fibrosis.

Management

Most of the patients with lichen sclerosis are obese, diabetic or thin fragile and anemic. In Bangladesh, these medical comorbidities often remain undiagnosed. Naturally, they need screening for diabetes mellitus, pernicious anemia and thyroid dysfunction. So, some investigations are required before going for actual treatment. Following investigations are helpful for the treatment of the patient:
- Blood sugar-fasting and two hours after 75 g of glucose.
- Serum thyroid stimulating hormone (TSH) and free thyroxine (FT4) level.
- Complete blood count.
- Serum iron, ferritin and total iron binding capacity (TIBC).
- Serum folic acid and vitamin B_{12} level.
- Many times the lesion is ulcerated and infected by multiple organisms. So, vulvar and vaginal swab may be collected for culture and sensitivity.

Treatment

Lichen sclerosus is treated by dermatologists, gynecologists, urologists and primary healthcare providers.[3]

Some general medical treatment needed to stop pruritus and to build up of epithelium. Medical treatments often needed are:
- Topical antibiotics should be given if the lesion is infected.
- Normal saline wash can be advised in place of soap, when the lesion is infected and dirty by necrosed tissue.

- Sometimes fungal infection flares up due to damage and tearing of the skin. So topical, antifungal cream is helpful in clearing up of infection and in building up of new epithelium.

General Advices to the Patient

- The patient should avoid tight undergarments, rubbing and scratching.
- Vulva should be kept clean by washing with water and mild soap, once or twice daily.
- Vulva should be kept dry and moisture less by proper aeration or using hair drier.
- If urine or fecal incontinence it should be treated.
- Emollient can be applied in the vulva to relieve dryness and itching and as a barrier to protect sensitive skin from contact with urine and feces.

Specific Medical Treatment

Local steroid therapy: Recent studies recommend treatment with very high potency steroid cream or ointment.[4,5] Lower potency topical steroids may be used in mild cases or when systemic therapy is contraindicated. Several regimens of steroid therapy can be used for the treatment of lichen sclerosis. Commonly used regimens are four. In all form of regimens, total duration of initial therapy is 12 weeks which is followed by maintenance therapy which is given as per requirement. Recommended four regimens are as follows:

- *Regimen 1 (one):* Clobetasol cream at the strength of 0.05% twice daily for 1 month and then once daily for 2 months. This regimen is found to be most effective with 75% success rate.
- *Regimen 2 (two):* Clobetasol cream 0.05% once at night for 4 weeks. At alternative night for 4 weeks. Then twice a week for 4 weeks.
- *Regimen 3 (three):* Clobetasol cream 0.05% twice daily for 6 weeks, then 1% betamethasone cream twice daily for 6 weeks.
- *Regimen 4 (four):* Clobetasol cream 0.05% twice daily for 12 weeks.

Then the dose is gradually lowered and tapered. Subsequent treatment with 0.05% clobetasol 2–3 times per weeks is used for maintenance therapy. Maintenance therapy can be continued as per need.

Patient is reviewed after 3 months of initiation of therapy. If symptom is resolved maintenance dose is continued. But if the symptoms persist or aggravate, topical steroid and topical retinoid (Vitamin A) therapy may be given.

Advices to the Patients during Treatment

- Patient is advised to come for follow-up if symptom does not improve after 1 month of use of clobetasol.
- A thin smear should be precisely applied to the white plaques and rubbed in gently.
- Itching often settles within a few days but it may take weeks to months for the skin to return to normal. One 30 g tube of topical steroid should last for 3–6 months.

Topical steroids are safe when used appropriately. However, excessive application to wrong sites can result in adverse effects in anogenital areas. Adverse effects which may be developed are

- Red, thin skin
- Burning vulva and vagina
- Periorificial dermatitis
- Superadded infections like *Candida albicans*.

It is most important for the patient to follow instructions carefully and to attend follow-up appointment regularly.

Other Topical Therapy

- Treatment with 2% testosterone cream, twice or three times daily for 6–12 weeks is also beneficial. But its long-term effectiveness may be less than that of clobetasol. Moreover, testosterone has potential unwanted side effects like virilization.
- Topical progesterone has also been used but its effectiveness is lacking.
- Topical low dose estrogen (1% estriol) therapy may be used. When lichen sclerosis is severe, acute or not responding to topical therapy systemic treatment may rarely be prescribed. Options are:
  - Intralesional or systemic corticosteroids-subcutaneous corticosteroid (e.g. triamcinolone acetonide suspension 10 mg/mL) injections have been used successfully. Hydroxyzine

hydrochloride can also be used at bed time to break the "itch-scratch" cycle.
- Oral retinoids
- Methotrexate
- Cyclosporine.

Surgery

Surgical excision should be considered in the following situations:
- Refractory cases
- Cases associated with high-grade squamous intraepithelial lesion or cancer
- Cases associated with vulval disfiguration
- Cases causing micturition, defecation or sexual difficulty.

Surgeries applicable for lichen sclerosis are:
- *Vulvar denervation (Mering procedure):* It can be considered when all other procedures are failed.
- *Alcohol injections:* Subcutaneous alcohol injections performed under general anesthesia interferes with the nerve endings and achieves relief for up to 6 months to a year.
- Laser ablation.
- Cryotherapy.
- Release of vulvar or vaginal adhesions and scarring may occasionally be performed to reduce urination difficulties and allow intercourse if dilators have not proved effective. Procedures include.
  - Simple perineotomy (division of adhesions)
  - Fenton's procedure in which an incision is given to release the adhesion and repaired transversely.
  - Perineoplasty which includes excision of involved vulval tissue and vaginal mucosal advancement.

Unfortunately, though after initial surgery has appeared successful, ultimately it recurs. But surgery can be done repeatedly.

Other Treatments

These are experimental and include:
- Phototherapy
- Photodynamic therapy

- Fat injections
- Stem cell and platelet-rich plasma injection.

Treatment success should be based on symptomatic improvement of pruritus, pain, dysuria and dyspareunia.

SQUAMOUS CELL HYPERPLASIA

The term squamous hyperplasia, with or without atypia, has been applied to proliferating epithelial lesions of the vulva. Such a term seems more meaningful to the clinician because it provides a point of reference compared to other proliferations in the cervix and endometrium. Typical hyperplastic dystrophy (squamous hyperplasia without atypia) corresponds to the classic picture of chronic dermatitis with hyperkeratosis. The epithelium is proliferated and there is acanthosis but no cellular atypia and no abnormal maturation. There is no malignant potential of this lesion.[6]

This benign epithelial and hyperkeratosis may be the result of chronic vulvovaginal infections or other causes of chronic irritations. Vulvar squamous cell hyperplasia is known by various names like:
- Hyperplastic dystrophy
- Leukoplakia
- Atopic dermatitis
- Atopic eczema
- Neurodermatitis.

The condition represents about 40–45% of the patients with non-neoplastic inflammatory vulvar epithelial disorders. Approximately two-thirds of the patients are premenopausal.

Squamous cell hyperplasia is not a distinct entity, it is only a description of a morphologic alteration of vulvar skin. Since the causes of vulvar epithelial hyperplasia are many, each of them should be properly identified, diagnosed and treated accordingly. Such conditions are:
- Lichen sclerosus
- Psoriasis
- Lichen planus
- Lichen simplex chronicus
- Vulvar eczema
- Seborrheic dermatosis

- Human papillomavirus infection
- Candida infection.

Squamous cell hyperplasia is a benign epithelial thickening and hyperkeratosis may be the result of above-mentioned chronic vulvovaginal infections and other causes of irritation.

The skin of the vulvar area is particular permeable to water in respect to the skin of other body sites. In this way, the vulvar region is moist and prone to absorb many compounds which occasionally come in the area. Almost any irritative condition may lead to hyperplastic changes. Among the factors implicated in the pathogenesis of hyperplasia, we can recognize intrinsic (physiologic sweat, psychogenic sweat, psychogenic pruritus, pruritus as the result of systemic disease) and extrinsic factors (physical, mechanical and chemical factors).

Presentation

Common presentation of the patients is pruritus. Itching, scrubbing and scratching are consequences of this initial event. This contributes to sustain and promote the circle leading to squamous cell hyperplasia.

Clinical Sign

Squamous cell hyperplasia is characterized by pink-red and moist vulva with overlying gray-white keratin. Areas most frequently involved are the prepuce, labia majora, interlabial sulci, outer aspect of the labia minora and the posterior commissure. The lesion may extend to the adjacent thighs. The size of the lesion is variable. The lesion may be macerated, raised, diffuse white or circumscribed.

Diagnosis

Diagnosis always needs histopathological examination of multiple punch biopsy specimen. Microscopic findings consist of:
- Elongation or widening of the rete ridges.
- Irregular thickening of the Malpighian layer of rete ridges (acanthosis).
- Hyperkeratosis.
- Chronic inflammatory cell infiltration in the dermis.

These are all nonspecific dermatological features that may be found in many pathological vulvar conditions. Then recent change in the nomenclature points out to describe squamous cell hyperplasia when other causes of hyperplastic epithelial changes are excluded on the basis of specific anatomical clinical features.

Treatment

Established hyperplastic vulvar dystrophy is not curable. Symptoms are variable and there may be long periods of remission. The severity of discomfort is also variable and depends on the degree of inflammation. Treatment of squamous cell hyperplasia is to reduce associated inflammation.

The relief of itching seems to be the first aim of any therapy. Itching can be relieved by improving vulvar skin hygiene. Following measures need to be taken for the relief of habit of itching:

- Identification and removal of any chemicals or moistures.
- Wearing white, cotton, loose underclothing.
- Avoiding rubbing with cloths.
- Frequent change of pads during menstruation.
- Use of dilute potassium permanganate wash, 2–3 times a day may have a vulvar skin soothing effect.
- Habit of rubbing and scrubbing by cloth can be relieved by giving oral antihistamine.
- If symptom of anxiety and irritability be present, oral tranquillizers at bed time may be used.

Mainstay of treatment for squamous cell hyperplasia is to prescribe topical medium potency corticosteroids. Betamethasone cream 0.1% twice daily for 2 weeks, then episodically is usually effective. If the vulvar skin is extremely thickened and an extensive lesion is found, a high potency (class I) steroid clobetasol propionate 0.05% twice daily for two weeks followed by betamethasone 0.05% when symptoms improves is effective. Care should be taken to avoid rebound effects of high potency clobetasol. The patient should be checked at close intervals and therapy switched to less potent steroid as soon as the symptomatology starts to improve. Steroid therapy for hyperplastic vulvar dystrophy does not need any maintenance therapy. But long-term surveillance is recommended. Refractory lesions may need intralesional injection of triamcinolone acetonide. Surgery should be avoided by all means because recurrence rate is 40–50%.

Malignant Potential

The risk of development of invasive cancer for women treated for squamous cell hyperplasia without intraepithelial neoplasia is minimal. It has been found that women with squamous cell hyperplasia occurring in a background of lichen sclerosus constitute a distinct group at higher risk of developing invasive cancer and require histologic assessment.

LICHEN PLANUS

Lichen planus of the vulva is part of the systemic manifestation of the skin and mucous membrane of other parts of the body. It is a unique inflammatory cutaneous and mucous membrane reaction of unknown etiology. This dermatological disorder may be associated with similar type of lesion at glabrous skin, hair-bearing skin and scalp and the mucous membrane of the oral cavity. The oral lesions are characterized by interlacing white lines on an erythematous mucosa. On the skin, the lesions are very small, polygonal, glistening papules that frequently have central umbilication. This is an uncommon cutaneous disease, probably autoimmune in origin and may rarely affect the vulva. Typical complains of vulvar lichen planus are vulvar burning and sometimes pruritus. The age range of the affected women is approximately 30–60 years. 10% of the patients may have a family history.

Clinical Signs

Labia minora and the vestibule are typically involved, the vagina can also be affected.
Typical clinical examination findings are:
- Ulceration and white patches in both the oral and vaginal/vulvar mucous membrane.
- Erythema and atrophy may be present.
- Ulceration may lead to coaptation of the labia with obliteration of the introitus (Fig. 2.5A).

Lichen planus is frequently misdiagnosed as atrophic or infectious vulvovaginitis. When conventional treatment is unsuccessful, a biopsy

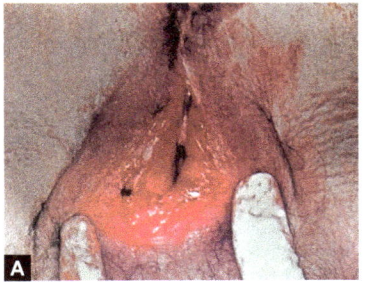 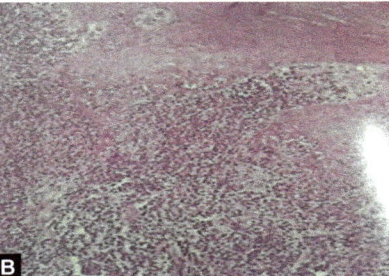

Figs. 2.5A and B: Lichen planus. (A) Ulceration of the labia. (B) Microscopic appearance showing lichen planus.

should be taken for correct diagnosis. The histopathological findings are:
- Acanthosis
- Basal cell degeneration with necrotic keratinocytes
- Heavy, band like lymphocytic and histiocytic infiltrate in the adjacent dermis (Fig. 2.5B).

If biopsy is taken from an area of ulceration or erosion, the epithelium will be absent and diagnosis of chronic ulcerative vulvitis is made. Treatment is with topical and systemic corticosteroids. But it has limited success.

Some patients have been successfully treated with subcutaneous injections of triamcinolone acetonamide suspension (10 mg/mL).[7] The main eruption clears within 1 year in 68% cases, but in 49% patients may have recurrence.

REFERENCES

1. DermNet NZ. (2016). All about the Skin. [online] Available from: http://www.dermnetnz.org/immune/lichen-sclerosus.html. [Accessed April, 2018].
2. British Association of Dermatologists. Lichen sclerosus in females. London: British Association of Dermatologists; 2014.
3. What is lichen sclerosus? Fast Facts: An Easy-to-Read Series of Publications for the Public. Washington: US Department of Health and Human Services Public Health Service; 2016.

4. Bracco GL, Carli P, Sonni L, et al. Clinical and histologic effects of topical treatments of vulval lichen sclerosus: a critical evaluation. J Reprod Med. 1993;38.37-40.
5. Carli P, Bracco, G, Taddei G, et al. Vulvar lichen sclerosus: immunohistologic evaluation before and after therapy. J Reprod Med. 1994:39:110-4.
6. Trimble CL, Trimble EL, Woodruff JD. Diseases of the vulva. In: Atkinson H (Ed). Clinical Gynecologic Pathology. Philadelphia: WB Saunders Company; 1996.p.36.
7. Trimble CL, Trimble EL, Woodruff JD. Diseases of the vulva. In: Atkinson H (Ed). Clinical Gynecologic Pathology. Philadelphia: WB Saunders Company; 1996.p.11.

CHAPTER 3

Non-neoplastic Inflammatory and Ulcerative Vulvar Disease

VULVAR VESTIBULITIS

It is a relatively common disorder of vulva. It is a condition of non-infective inflammatory disorder of the vestibule of vulva. Complaints of the patient are characterized by vulvar pain and severe acquired entry dyspareunia. Slightly erythematous, tender macules are found in the mucosa of the vestibule (Fig. 3.1). The lesion commonly involves the

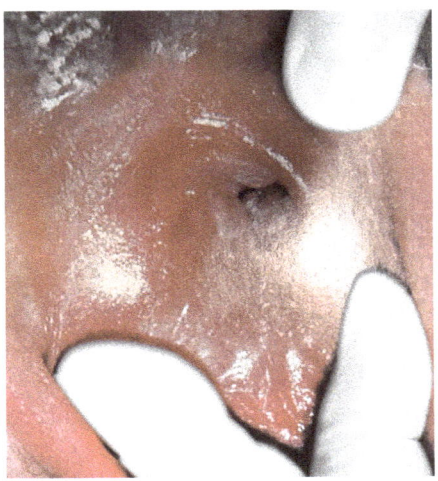

Fig. 3.1: Vulvar vestibulitis syndrome.

fourchette. Biopsy shows a nonspecific chronic inflammatory infiltrate in the subepithelial stroma surrounding the minor vestibular glands. The etiology is not known. Perineoplasty offers the best treatment results. By this surgical procedure symptomatic improvement occurs in one-third of the patients.[1,2]

VULVAR PSORIASIS

The mons and crural folds are relatively common sites of psoriasis; however, the vulva is rarely the sole site of involvement on the body. The gross appearance of psoriasis on the vulva is often atypical and frequently does not resemble psoriasis elsewhere. The characteristics "silver scales" of psoriasis are often absent in the vulva owing to the moisture in the area. Nevertheless the classic features are usually apparent on lesions elsewhere on the body. The lesions are irregular, multifocal patches that have an erythematous background. Elevated silver scales may be prominent. The adjacent skin may demonstrate excoriations, accentuation of the skin markings, or lichenification.

FOX–FORDYCE DISEASE

Fox–Fordyce disease is caused by obstruction of the apocrine gland. The labia majora and mons are dotted with tiny, slightly elevated, firm, intensely pruritic papules (Fig. 3.2A). The labia minora, prepuce, and clitoris, which do not contain apocrine glands, are spared in this disease, but these areas may be edematous (Fig. 3.2B). On microscopic examination focal nests of dilated apocrine glands are found that show little, if any, evidence of inflammatory reaction (Fig. 3.2C). The process is usually cyclic and is related to the secretary activity of the apocrine glands. Oral contraceptives (which reduce apocrine gland secretions) and local antipruritic medications are usually effective.

CROHN'S DISEASE

Crohn's disease, also known as regional enteritis may involve the lower genital tract. Draining sinuses and rectoperianal or rectovaginal fistula develop in approximately 20–25% of patients with documented intestinal disease.[3,4] These may drain into the posterior fourchette. The adjacent vulva may show linear excoriations and edema (Fig. 3.3).

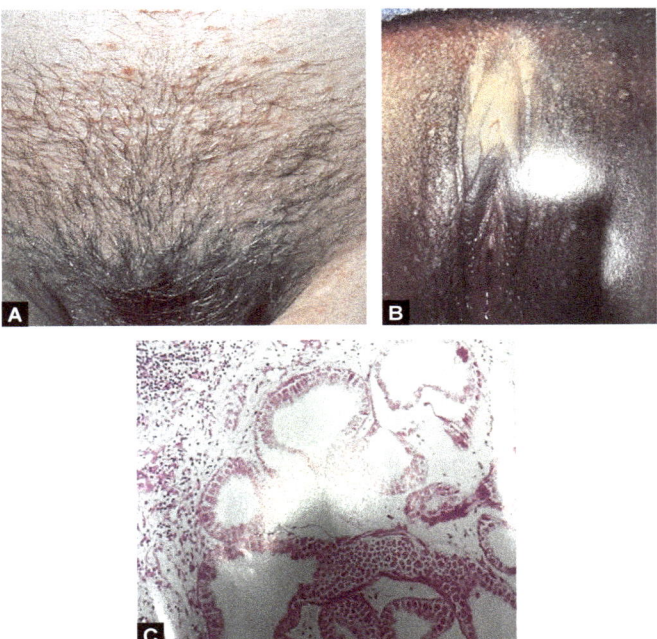

Figs. 3.2A to C: Fox-Fordyce disease. (A) Labia majora and mons are dotted with tiny and pruritic papules. (B) Affected labia minora, prepuce, and clitoris. (C) Microscopic examination shows evidence of inflammatory reaction.

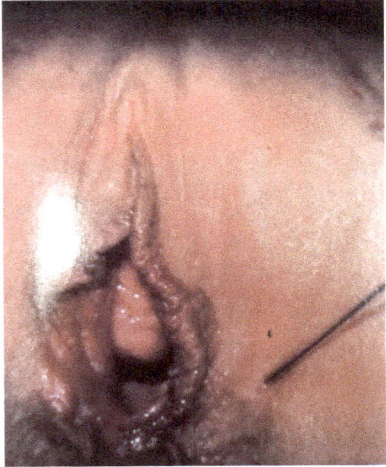

Fig. 3.3: Crohn's disease.

The diagnosis is difficult unless the clinician is aware of the condition and its association on rare occasions, there may be little or no definite evidence of intestinal Crohn disease. Biopsy of the lesion from intestine or from the fistula tract shows a chronic inflammatory infiltrate and occasionally noncaseating granulomas may be present.

Treatment consists of preoperative systemic steroids and metronidazole followed by surgery. Surgery is done to remove the granulation tissue and repair of fistula. Without these perioperative medications, surgery is doomed to fail.

BEHCET SYNDROME

Behcet disease or syndrome is characterized by a triad of recurrent aphthous ulcerations in the mouth (Fig. 3.4) and on the vulva that are associated with inflammatory vacuities of the eye. Any one or all three of these components may be present, but uveitis is less frequent than vulvar and oral ulcerations. The patients with Behcet disease may also experience meningoencephalitis, recurrent synovitis, cutaneous pustules or nodules resembling erythema nodosum, phlebitis of large and small veins, arterial aneurysms in the systemic and pulmonary circulation and discrete gastrointestinal ulcers that can bleed or perforate.

An acute ulcer of Behcet disease is sharply marginated and has a grayish-white necrotic center when it occurs in the mouth. On the

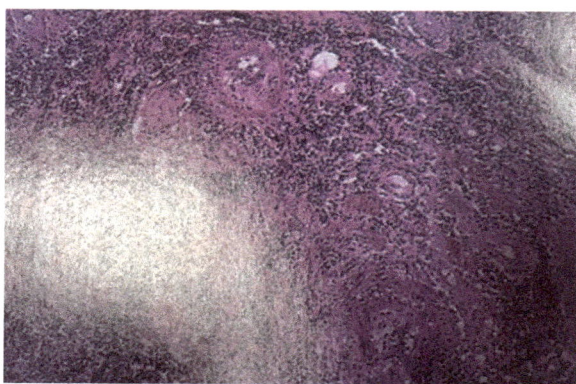

Fig. 3.4: Behcet's syndrome.

vulva it may be reddish-yellow. Surprisingly, these ulcers may produce no symptoms. In the chronic phase distortion of the labia with tissue fenestrations may develop. Biopsy in the chronic phase shows an intense mucosal and submucosal chronic inflammatory infiltrates with accompanying florid vasculitis, which culminates in occlusion of the submucosal vessels.

The cause of the disease is unknown, but vasculitis is the key factor in the pathogenesis. An autoimmune process has been suggested.[5] The clinical diagnosis is frequently one exclusion after other destructive lesions affecting the vulva, such as Crohn disease, pemphigus, herpes, and syphilis, have been excluded. The lesions are usually self-limiting and thus the effectiveness of various therapies is difficult to assess. Fatal cases are almost always associated with eye lesions and involvement of the central nervous system. Interesting thing is the reported association of exacerbations with menstrual cycle. Improvement with the use of oral contraceptives has noted. This may be coincidental and be related to the frequent spontaneous exacerbations and regressions for which this disease is noted. Systemic corticosteroid treatment is the most widely used effective therapy.[6]

Aphthous Ulcers

Aphthous ulcers occur in the vulvar area where they are usually asymptomatic. These are shallow ulcers that are probably caused by trauma. No treatment is necessary because spontaneous healing is rapid. A topical anesthetic can be used if the lesion is painful. If the lesion does not heal, biopsy is mandatory to exclude a malignant disease (Figs. 3.5A and B).

Other Ulcers

Pemphigus vulgaris, Darier disease (keratosis follicularis), and Hailey-Hailey disease (familial benign chronic pemphigus) can also involve the vulva. Biopsy, which is mandatory for all ulcerative lesions of the vulva, demonstrates acantholysis in patients with pemphigus. This is the process of disintegration of the intercellular bridges between the keratinocytes, which leads to an intraepidermal cleft or bulla. The superficial epithelium is separated from the first two three cell layers of

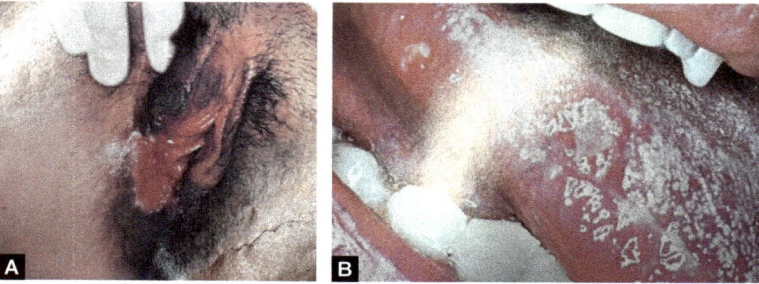

Figs. 3.5A and B: Aphthous ulcers—(A) Vulva, (B) Mouth.

the basal zone. Acantholytic cells line the bulla and also lie free within the cavity of the bulla. These cells have a large basophilic nucleus that may be surrounded by a clear halo. Moderate hyperkeratosis is seen over the bulla.

Finally, it should be noted that both decubitus and factitious (self-induced) ulcerations may be present on the vulva as in other locations on the baby. The former are usually self-evident and occur most frequently in patients with poor circulation. Factitious ulcers present a clinical rather than a histopathological challenge because the psychological aspects of the problem may be bizarre and difficult to characterize.

SYSTEMIC DISEASE

The vulva, like the skin elsewhere, may reflect the presence of systemic disease. A patient who has poorly controlled diabetes mellitus may complain of vulvar pruritus. This usually due to an infection with *Candida albicans*. In the acute phase there is intense erythema of the labia minora and majora and satellite erythematous lesions that involve the intracrural folds and inner thighs (Fig. 3.6A). In the chronic phase of candidal infection hyperkeratosis is present. On physical examination thickened and grayish epithelium is found, interspersed by small superficial reddish areas (Fig. 3.6B). Excoriations from scratching are usually present. A dramatic response to topical antifungal agents and control of the diabetes is seen.

Chronic anemia is occasionally accompanied by vulvar ulceration. Uremic frost may be appreciated as brownish-yellow patches on the

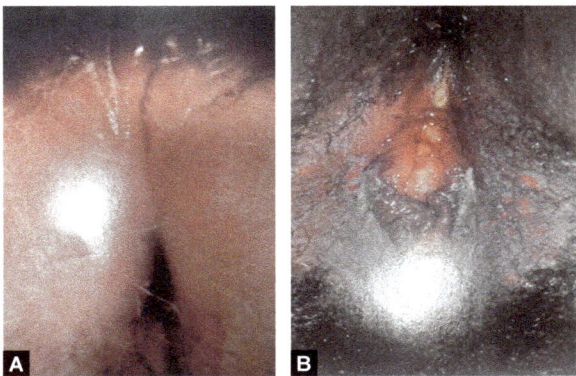

Figs 3.6A and B: Acute and chronic phases of systemic disease.

vulva. Systemic sarcoidosis may present on the vulva as grayish-white thickened skin. This is due to hyperkeratosis, which is characteristic of most chronic inflammatory conditions of the vulva. Biopsy reveals noncaseating granulomas with multiple giant cells seen in the dermis. These may be seen in many other conditions, and the diagnosis of sarcoidosis depends on their presence at other more typical sites including the lung, lymph nodes, and liver and the lack of infectious agents or other diseases such as Crohn's disease.

REFERENCES

1. Scurry J, Dennerstein G, Brenan J, et al. Vulvitis circumscripta plasmacellularis: a clinicopathologic entity? J Reprod Med. 1993;38:14-8.
2. Friedrich EG. Vulvar vestibulitis syndrome. J Reprod Med. 1987;32:110-4.
3. Donalson LB. Crohn's disease: its gynaecologic aspect. Am J Obstet Gynecol. 1978;131:196-202.
4. Kremer M, Nussenson E, Steinfeld M, et al. Crohn's disease of the vulva. Am J Gestroenterol. 1984;79:376-8.
5. O' Duffy JD. Behcet's syndrome. N Engl J Med. 1990;322:326-7.
6. Wong RC, Ellis CN, Diaz LA. Behcet's disease: a review. Int J Dermatol. 1984;23:25-32.

CHAPTER 4

Vulvar Intraepithelial Neoplasia

INTRODUCTION

Vulvar intraepithelial neoplasia (VIN) is an increasingly common problem, particularly among women in their 40s. Like cervical intraepithelial neoplasia (CIN), premalignant condition of vulva is called vulvar intraepithelial neoplasia.

Vulvar skin is one of the components of anogenital epithelium. The lower genital tract epithelium is of common cloacogenic origin. Neoplasia of vulvar skin is often associated with multiple foci of dysplasia in the lower genital tract.

Vulvar intraepithelial neoplasia is defined as dysplastic changes in the vulvar squamous epithelium characterized by the presence of immature cells, cellular disorganization and increased mitotic activity as in CIN changes of the cervix and vaginal intraepithelial neoplasia (VAIN) changes of the vagina.

INCIDENCE AND ETIOLOGY

Since 1970s, marked increase in incidence of high-grade VIN and a decrease in modal age of diagnosis has been observed. Surveillance, Epidemiology and End Results (SEER) data from the United States have shown a four-fold increase in diagnosis of VIN between 1973 and 2000.[1] However, the incidence of vulvar carcinoma has remained relatively constant presumably because the preinvasive disease is actively treated.

Although 85% of high grade VIN lesions are human papilloma virus associated, human papillomavirus (HPV) DNA is detected only in approximately 40% of vulvar cancers. Many of the HPV negative cancers, particularly in older women are associated with lichen sclerosus.[2] HPV type 16 is commonly associated with VIN. 50% VIN is associated with CIN or VAIN and 20–30% is associated with invasive squamous cell carcinoma of vulva. The risk of malignant transformation of VIN is 3–12%. It takes less than 8 years to change to invasive cancer.

A strong association exists between sexually transmitted disease and high grade of VIN particularly VIN-3. Primarily HPV, but also gonorrhea, syphilis, gardnerella vaginalis, trichomoniasis are associated with VIN which rates varying from 20% to 60%. Other risk factors include smoking, immunosuppressive disease, radiation therapy, pregnancy and other genital precancers and cancers. VIN can be viral or nonviral etiology. Young women are more commonly affected by viral VIN than older women and also are more likely to exhibit multifocal disease. In older women, the lesion is usually unifocal and arises de novo.

RELATION BETWEEN VULVAR DYSTROPHY, VIN AND INVASIVE SQUAMOUS CELL CARCINOMA VULVA

Vulvar intraepithelial neoplasia has traditionally been considered to be premalignant condition, and to be one disease, but in 2004, the International Society for the Study of Vulvovaginal Disease (ISSVD) officially divided VIN in to two types: (1) usual type VIN, which is related to HPV infection, and (2) differentiated type VIN, which is unrelated to HPV infection (Box 4.1).[3] The term VIN I is no longer used, and VIN 2 and VIN 3 are simply called VIN.

The older classification of VIN 1, 2, and 3 was based on the degree of histologic abnormality, but there is no evidence that the VIN 1 to 3 morphologic spectrum reflects a biologic continuum, or that VIN 1 is a cancer precursor.[3]

It is now generally accepted that there are two different etiologic types of vulvar cancer. One type is seen mainly in younger patients, is related to HPV infection and smoking, and is commonly associated

> **BOX 4.1:** Squamous vulvar intraepithelial neoplasia (VIN) [2004 International Society for the Study of Vulvar Disease (ISSVD) Terminology].
>
> I. VIN, usual type
>   a. VIN, warty type
>   b. VIN, basaloid type
>   c. VIN, mixed (warty/basaloid) type
> II. VIN, differentiated type
>
> *Source:* Reproduced with permission from Sideri M, Jones RW, Wilkinson EJ, et al. Squamous vulvar intraepithelial neoplasia: 2004 modified terminology, ISSVD Vulvar Oncology Subcommittee. J Reprod Med. 2005;50:807-10.

with basaloid or warty VIN. The more common type is seen mainly in elderly patients, is unrelated to smoking or HPV infection, and concurrent VIN is uncommon. There is, however, a high incidence of dystrophic lesions, including lichen sclerosus and squamous hyperplasia, adjacent to the tumor. If VIN is present, it is of the differentiated type.

Using data on 2,685 patients with invasive vulvar cancer from the National Cancer Institute's Surveillance Epidemiology and End Results program (SEER), Sturgeon et al. reported the increased risk of a subsequent cancer to be 1.3-fold. Most of the second cancers were related to smoking (i.e. cancers of the lung, buccal cavity, pharynx, nasal cavity, or larynx) or to infection with human papillomavirus (e.g. cervix vagina, or anus).[4]

In a study designed to investigate the malignant potential of the vulvar premalignant conditions, Eva et al. identified 580 women from Birmingham, England, who had vulvar biopsies showing VIN, lichen sclerosus, or squamous hyperplasia over a 5-year period.[5] These women were studied for the presence of a synchronous of metachronous vulvar cancer. The authors reported that differentiated VIN had a higher risk of malignancy (85.7%) than usual VIN (25.8%), lichen sclerosus (27.7%) or squamous hyperplasia (31.7%).

Dutch workers between 1992 and 2005 in their prospective study, found that the malignant potential of premalignant conditions to be much lower 5.7% for usual VIN, 32% for differential VIN, and 2-6% for lichen sclerous.[6]

Patients with lichen sclerosus and concomitant hyperplasia may be at risk for malignant transformation. Rodke et al. reported development of vulvar carcinoma in 3 of 18 such cases (17%), postulating that areas of hyperplasia were superimposed on a background of lichen sclerosus because of chronic irritation and trauma.[7]

Carli et al. from the vulvar clinic at the University of Florence, Italy, reported an association with lichen sclerosus in 32% of their cases of vulvar cancer that were not HPV related.[8] They felt that the existence of accessory conditions necessary to promote the progression from lichen sclerosus to cancer remained to be established. Scurry believes lichen sclerosus contributes to a vicious cycle of itching and scratching, which leads to superimposed lichen simplex chronicus, squamous cell hyperplasia, and ultimately carcinoma.[9]

CLASSIFICATION OF VULVAR INTRAEPITHELIAL NEOPLASIA

Traditionally, squamous vulvar intraepithelial neoplasia was classified into three grades, analogous to the three-grade CIN classification. Preinvasive neoplasia of the vulva has been recognized for more than 75 years, but the descriptive terminology has been confusing. The degree of loss of epithelial cellular maturation in a given lesion defines the grade of VIN. Histologically VIN has been graded as:

- VIN I or mild dysplasia where dysplastic changes are found in lower one-third of the vulvar epithelium.
- VIN II or moderate dysplasia where dysplastic cells are found in lower two-thirds of the vulvar epithelium.
- VIN III or severe dysplasia where dysplastic cells are found in more than lower two-thirds of the vulvar epithelium.

When whole thickness epithelium is involved by dysplastic changes it is called vulvar carcinoma in situ (CIS). Microscopically essential features of vulvar CIS is the absence of penetration of basement membrane. Vulvar CIS has been described as Bowen's disease, erythroplasia of Queyrat, CIS simplex, Bowenoid papulosis or kraurosis vulvae and leukoplakia. Bowen's disease is applied to some cases of VIN when large Bowen's cells, sometimes corp rords appear in the malignant cell. Bowen's cells are large cells with perinuclear vacuolation and nuclear fragmentation. It is usually found in association with HPV infection.

Current Classification of VIN

Subsequent studies determined that VIN 1 reflects usually a self-limited infection caused by human papillomavirus (HPV). In 2004, the ISSVD replaced the previous three-grade classification system with the current single-grade system, in which only high-grade disease is classified as VIN.[10] In the current system, VIN is subdivided into usual-type VIN (including warty, basaloid, and mixed VIN) and differentiated VIN. Usual-type VIN is commonly associated with carcinogenic genotypes of HPV and other HPV persistence risk factors, such as cigarette smoking and immunocompromised status, whereas differentiated VIN usually is not associated with HPV and is more often associated with vulvar dermatologic conditions, such as lichen sclerosus. However, differentiated VIN associated with lichen sclerosus is more likely to be associated with a squamous cell carcinoma of the vulva than usual-type VIN.

Flat lesions associated with basal atypia and koilocytic changes (formerly termed VIN 1) are considered condylomas in the current ISSVD classification system and can be treated as such.[10] Other intraepithelial vulvar neoplasms, such as Paget's disease and melanoma in situ, are rare.

NATURAL HISTORY OF VULVAR INTRAEPITHELIAL NEOPLASIA

There is some basis for establishing a biological continuum from CIN I to CIN III. But the neoplastic biologic continuum from VIN I through VIN III to invasive cancer had not been established.

Although the progression rate of VIN III to invasive cancer remains controversial, the malignant potential has been established. By contrast, there is no direct evidence that VIN I has any malignant potential.

There is compelling argument for excluding low-grade VIN from the "intraepithelial neoplasia" category.[11] When mild squamous atypia is seen in vulvar skin, usually limited to lower epidermis, the lesion is more likely to be non-neoplastic reactive atypia. Considerable interobserver and intraobserver variation occurs with the VIN I diagnosis and this diagnostic category is not reproducible.[10]

Most histologic VIN lesions are categorized as VIN 2-3 and good histologic agreement is obtained when VIN-II and VIN-III are combined as a single high-grade VIN diagnose.[10] Only 10-15% of VIN is not associated with any coexistent disease. It coexists with invasive lesion in 30-50% of cases. Lichen sclerosus and hypertrophic type vulvar dystrophy occurs in 50% of the specimen. One report made by Jones and Rowan from New Zealand in 1994 on follow-up of 113 women with VIN III diagnosed between 1961 and 1993. Among eight untreated cases of VIN III, there was progression to invasive cancer in seven patients (87%) within 8 years. This risk may be as high as 100% for women over 40. Another recent study from New Zealand reported spontaneous regression of VIN II-III.[12] These women were young (medical age 24 years) with sexually transmitted disease. Most had multifocal pigmented lesion and median time to regression was 9.5 months.

TERMINOLOGY FOR SQUAMOUS VULVAR INTRAEPITHELIAL NEOPLASIA

In 2004, the ISSVD recommended the following modifications to the terminology for squamous vulvar intraepithelial neoplasia.[10]
1. The VIN I should no longer be used, being replaced with the terms flat condyloma acuminatum or HPV effect. The term "atypia" in this context is discouraged.
2. The term VIN should apply to histologic high-grade squamous intraepithelial lesions (VIN 2-3).
3. Two categories of VIN were described:
   a. The more common VIN, usual type, which enocompasses VIN 2, VIN 3, and the older clinical and histologic terms: Bowen's disease, bowenoid papulosis, dysplasia, and CIS. These lesions are associated with high-risk HPV types, particularly HPV 16. VIN, usual type, has been subcategorized histologically as warty (condylomatous), basaloid, or mixed.
   b. The less-common VIN, differentiated type. These lesions are not associated with HPV, but frequently occur against a background of a dermatosus, particularly lichen sclerosus.
4. The occasional VIN lesion that cannot be classified as VIN, usual or differentiated types is termed VIN, unclassified type (or VIN, NOS). (This includes the rare pagetoid VIN).

> **BOX 4.2:** International Society for the Study of Vulvar Disease (ISSVD) classification of vulvar diseases.
>
> 1. *Non-neoplastic epithelial disorders of skin and mucosa of vulva*
>   – Lichen sclerosus (formerly lichen sclerosus et atrophicus)
>   – Squmous hyperplasia (formerly hyperplastic dystrophy)
>   – Other dermatoses (e.g. psoriasis)
> 2. *Intraepithelial neoplasia*
>   – Squamous intraepithelial neoplasia
>   ◆ VIN, usual type
>   - VIN, warty type
>   - VIN, basaloid type
>   - VIN, mixes (warty/basaloid) type
>   ◆ VIN, differentiated type
>   – Nonsquamous intraepithelial neoplasia
>   ◆ Paget's disease
>   ◆ Tumors of the melanocytes, noninvasive (melanoma in situ)
> 3. Mixed non-neoplastic and neoplastic epithelial disorders
> 4. Invasive tumors
>
> (VIN: Vulvar intraepithelial neoplasia)
> *Source:* International Society for the Study of Vulvar Disease (Committee on Terminology, 2004).

5. Classification is on the basis of histologic morphology only, and clinical appearance or HPV type. The 2004 ISSVD classification of VIN is shown in Box 4.2.

CLINICAL PROFILE OF VULVAR SQUAMOUS INTRAEPITHELIAL NEOPLASIA

The increasing incidence of VIN 3 in recent decades reflects increased clinical awareness, improved diagnostic accuracy and an absolute increase in disease incidence. Symptom distribution of VIN lesion in younger and older women is variable. The lesion is commonly localized and unifocal in older patients, which is usually not associated with HPV infection. Malignant potential in these women are higher, because invasive vulvar cancer occurs in older age group.

In younger, the lesion tends to be multifocal and extensive. The size of the lesion varies from several mm to large confluent lesion involving the whole vulva. It may remain as small discrete lesion or multiple lesion coalesce to develop a large lesion.

Common sites involved are non-hair bearing areas of the vulva extending laterally from labia majora to the hair-bearing skin of the labia majora and anteroposteriorly from mons pubis to posterior fourchette, perineum and perianal skin.

Appearance of the VIN lesions vary in color from white to black, red, gray or brown depending on the age, race and complexion of the patient.

White Lesion

The lesion may be raised, papular or flat macular type. Usually papular lesion occurs at the keratinized skin and flat macular lesion occurs at the mucosal surface. Macular lesions are subclinical and are detected on colposcopic examination after application of 5% acetic acid solution.

White lesions occur as a result of hyperkeratosis or dehydration of the outer keratinized layer. Red lesion results from increased vascularity, secondary to inflammatory response or due to angiogenetic factors of neoplasia. Brown or pigmented lesion result from pigmented melanin deposition (Figs. 4.1 to 4.3).

Symptoms

Majority are asymptomatic, only 30% with VIN III experience some vulvar symptoms, mostly pruritus, vulvar irritation and burning, pain and dysuria. The symptoms are exacerbated by voiding. Other complains may be:
- Localized lump or swelling
- Thickening of vulvar skin
- Area of altered pigmentation

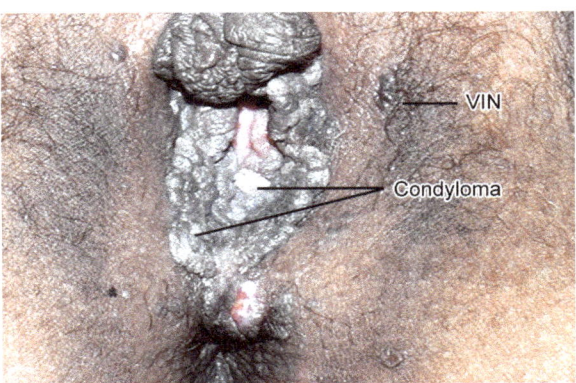

Fig. 4.1: Patient with multiple condyloma and vulvar intraepithelial neoplasia (VIN).

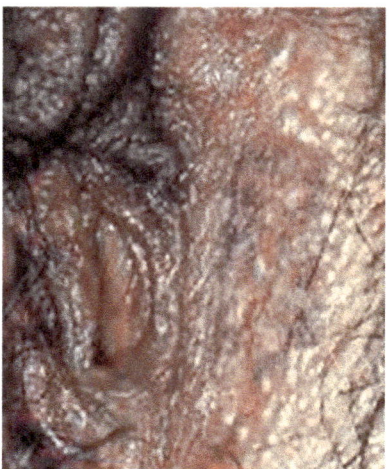

Fig. 4.2: Hyperpigmented vulvar intraepithelial neoplasia (VIN)—usual type.

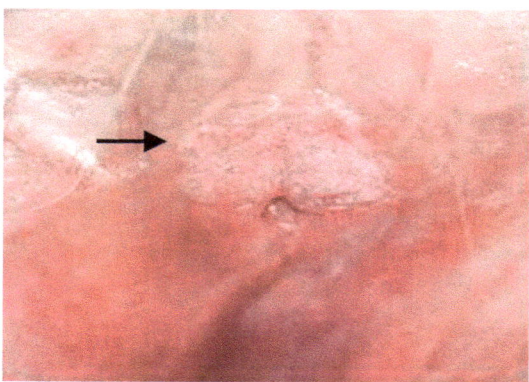

Fig. 4.3: Vulvar intraepithelial neoplasia showing warty growth.

- Change in color
- Dyspareunia
- Difficulty in voiding stool.

Microscopic Appearance

The microscopic appearance of vulvar squamous intraepithelial lesion is characterized by:
- Cellular disorganization
- Loss of stratification

- Increased cellular density
- Great variation in cell size
- Presence of giant multinucleated cell
- Hypercromatism
- HPV-related cytopathy such as perinuclear halos with displacement of nucleus are also common. Essential feature is the absence of penetration of basement membrane (Fig. 4.4).

Diagnosis

Vulvar intraepithelial neoplasia is a multifocal disease, especially in young women, when it is caused by HPV infection. Possibly 1-2% of young women with cervical dysplasia will be found to have involve the upper third of the vagina and the vulva, perineum and perianal area as these surfaces arise from a common cloacogenic origin. A spectrum of diseases ranging from mild dysplasia to carcinoma in situ may be found in the same lesion.

No screening strategies have been developed for the prevention of vulvar cancer through early detection of VIN. Vulvar cytological testing is complicated by the keratinization of vulvar skin, making performance and interpretation of test results problematic. Diagnosis is limited to visual assessment. Clinically VIN lesion is quite variable. Most women have visible lesions that are elevated, but flat lesions occur. Color can vary from white to gray or from red to brown to black. So, carefully naked eye inspection of the lesion is mandatory.

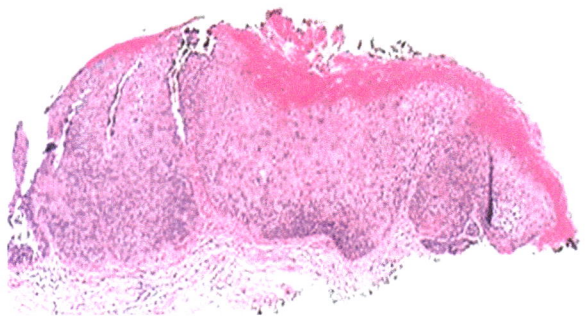

Fig. 4.4: Microscopic appearance of vulvar squamous intraepithelial lesion— absence of penetration of basement membrane.

Biopsy is indicated for any pigmented vulvar lesion. Expert opinion is derived regarding the need for biopsy of all warty lesions, but biopsy should be performed in postmenopausal women with apparent genital warts and in women in whom topical therapies have failed.

Colposcopic evaluation in higher magnification (6–7 times) with or without green filter may be helpful. An abnormal vascular pattern is most frequently associated with a severe degree of dysplasia, carcinoma in situ or early invasive disease. Nowadays colposcopy is an accepted standard procedure in the diagnostic assessment of VIN. Colposcopic examination, diagnosis of abnormal area and biopsy of any suspicious lesion is the gold standard for diagnosis of VIN. Although toluidine blue testing is often cited for use in the assessment of VIN, this method is infrequently used and rarely beneficial in the diagnosis of VIN.

Colposcopic Procedure

After application of 5% acetic acid solution and colposcopic assessment, lesions appear as clearly demarcated, dense acetowhite areas. The multifocal distribution is usually evident. The acetic acid reaction is seen in lesions that are nonpigmented or red. Pigmented lesions often develop an acetowhite hue or a rim of acetowhitening. Initial clinical examination may identify clinically apparent lesions. Colposcopy may permit identification of previously unidentified, subclinical lesions and better define the distribution of clinically evident disease.

In high-grade vulvar preinvasive lesions, vascular patterns are often inconspicuous or absent, particularly in the presence of hyperkeratosis. Macular lesions on the mucous membranes may reveal a capillary punctuation pattern, and a fine punctuation is sometimes observed in papular lesions. Marked vascular abnormalities characterized by a varicose, widely spaced punctuation and rarely, mosaicism represent a definite warning sign of invasive cancer and the lesion must be excised. Colposcopic warning signs of vulvar cancer occur late in the neoplastic process. Histologic evidence of VIN may be seen outside colposcopically identified margins of disease, particularly laterally in the hair-bearing areas.

Diagnosis ultimately depends on liberal use of directed biopsy. This is particularly the case if ablative treatment is being considered either alone or in combination with excisional procedures. *Biopsies are best taken with a Keyes biopsy instrument* under local anesthesia in the office setting.

Prevention

Immunization with the quadrivalent HPV vaccine, which is effective against HPV genotypes 6, 11, 16, and 18, has been shown to decrease the risk of VIN and should be recommended for women in target populations. The bivalent HPV vaccine is not approved for this indication, because this endpoint was not assessed in clinical trials. Cigarette smoking is strongly associated with usual-type VIN, and cessation should be encouraged, although no studies have shown a reduction in VIN incidence or post-treatment recurrence after smoking-cessation efforts. Differentiated VIN may be associated with vulvar dermatoses, and treatment of vulvar dermatologic disorders may reduce VIN and cancer risk.

Treatment

Treatment is recommended for all women with VIN. But in younger patients spontaneous regression may occur. So, there are some indications for observation for 6-12 months. Indications for observation are:
- When the patient is young with mild dysplasia and good compliance,
- Patients who have recently completed a course of corticosteroid therapy,
- Patients who were recently pregnant or were temporarily immunocompromised. These patients should be reviewed at every 3-6 months and if the disease is persistent or worse, then her treatment is indicated.

Aim of treatment of VIN:
- To give symptomatic relief.
- To rule out associated CIN, VAIN and invasive cancer of vulva.
- To rule out associated sexually transmitted disease.

- To choose the technique, which will give optimal result while preserving normal tissue and function.
- To prevent progression to invasive cancer.

Symptomatic Relief

Primary symptoms of VIN are pain and pruritus. Pain can be relieved by the use of various types of analgesics like nonsteroidal anti-inflammatory drugs (NSAIDs). Use of simple paracetamol can also be helpful. For relief of pruritus various types of antihistamine can be used. VIN can be associated with various types of sexually transmitted infections, including moniliasis, trichomoniasis, chlamydia infection, herpes simplex, lymphogranuloma venereum, granuloma inguinale, gonorrhea and syphilis, all of them cause various types of discharge. So, discharge needs to treat accordingly. To rule out associated CIN and VAIN Pap's smear should be done in all patients of VIN. Colposcopy is an essential tool to rule out CIN and VAIN. Sometimes anoscopy is needed if the anal margin is involved.

Treatment Options

Many treatment modalities have been used so far. And traditionally vulvar CIS has been treated by simple vulvectomy. Such a radical approach is unjustified as the procedure is associated with significant morbidity like scarring, dyspareunia, urinary stream difficulties, loss of elasticity for vaginal delivery. These problems are more painful in younger women.

Since 1970, more conservative approach has been tried. Nowadays treatment options for VIN are—(1) medical treatment and (b) surgical treatment.

Medical treatment can be offered to some older patients who are unfit for surgical treatment. Treatment is given by the use of 5-fluorouracil or bleomycin cream for 6–10 weeks. But this treatment by local chemotherapeutic agent may be associated with severe local inflammatory response after 2 weeks of use. When severe inflammatory response develops, treatment should be prematurely discontinued. Then the patient is treated symptomatically and when re-epithelialization occur which is expected within 4–6 weeks' time, treatment is restarted.

Medical therapy: Randomized controlled trials have shown that the application of topical imiquimod 5% is effective for the treatment of VIN, although it is not approved by the US Food and Drug Administration for this purpose.[13] Published regimens include three times weekly application to affected areas for 12-20 weeks, with colposcopic assessment at 4-6 week intervals during treatment. Residual lesions require surgical treatment. Erythema and vulvar pain may limit adverse effects. Experience with imiquimod in immunosuppressed patients is limited, and because it is believed to act through local immunomodulators, it may have decreased effectiveness in women who are immunocompromised.

Surgical treatment: Surgery remains the hallmark of treatment modality for VIN. Surgical treatment options are:
- Wide local excision
- Laser ablation
- Superficial vulvectomy (skinning vulvectomy) with or without split-thickness skin grafting.

Extent of surgery or surgical procedure depends on the extent of involvement of the vulva, perineum and perianal skin which should be defined by colposcopic evaluation.

Wide local excision: It is the preferred option for unifocal single lesion. Indications of this procedure are:
- When cancer is suspected clinically or pathologically.
- To obtain a specimen for pathologic reevaluation, despite a biopsy diagnosis of only VIN.
- Wide local excision is also acceptable in women in whom cancer is not suspected.
- It is mandatory if a lesion has warning sign of possible invasive cancer.

Excision of small unifocal lesion: The lesion should be excised with a disease free margin of at last 5 mm. For unifocal lesions, a 1 cm margin of uninvolved skin is usually curative. If the margins involved, the cure rate falls to 50%. Primary closure of the defect usually achieves uncomplicated healing with a very satisfactory cosmetic and functional outcome. Elasticity of the vulvar skin permits preservation of sexual and reproductive functions.

Surgical specimen should be submitted to careful histologic evaluation to exclude invasive disease and to ensure clean surgical margins. As long as all macroscopic disease has been removed, re-excision is not justified for microscopic positive margins. Most recurrences occur within 3 years of treatment, although late recurrence and progression to cancer can occur. Developments of symptom are the warning for prompt urgent review.

Excision of large confluent or multifocal disease: This type of extensive disease, particularly when associated with colposcopic warning signs of early invasion, require more extensive procedures with rotational flaps to fill the defect.

Primary closure of the wound may not be possible without under tension, leading to would breakdown or excessive screening. So, cutaneous or flaps with no muscle component have been used for these cases.

"Skinning" vulvectomy was introduced by Rutledge and Sinclair (1968) for extensive widespread multifocal VIN lesion of hair-bearing skin where the skin appendages may be involved.

Procedure: The lesions are clearly mapped and a shallow layer of vulvar skin is excised, preserving the subcutaneous tissues. Then a split-thickness skin grafting with epidermis from a donor site on the inner aspect of the thigh or buttock is done. The epithelium regenerates without loss of sensation.

Indications of skinning vulvectomy
- In young woman, it is advantageous to preserve the subcutaneous tissue.
- In immune compromised women, the disease is often confluent, multifocal.

Simple vulvectomy: In elderly women, as there is a need to exclude occult invasive disease or VIN in these old women may be associated with lichen sclerosus and often the lesions are not amenable to conservative therapy, so simple vulvectomy is indicated for them.

Laser ablation (AOCOG): Laser ablation is acceptable for the treatment of VIN when cancer is not suspected. It can be used for single, multifocal, or confluent lesions, although the risk of recurrence may be higher than with excision. Appropriate power density (750–1,250 W/cm^2) is critical to avoid deep coagulation injury.[14,15] Colposcopy after application of 3–5% acetic acid facilitates delineation of lesion margins, and use of a micromanipulator or a hand piece with a depth gauge allows application of high-power density without inadvertent defocusing. As with excision, a margin of normal-appearing skin should be treated. In contrast to its application to genital warts, when superficial ablation is acceptable, laser treatment of VIN requires destruction of cells through the entire thickness of the epithelium. In hair-bearing areas, laser procedures must ablate hair follicles, which can contain VIN and extend into the subcutaneous fat for 3 mm or more. Consequently, large VIN lesions over hair-bearing areas may be preferentially treated with other modalities. Ablation over skin that does not bear hair should extend through the dermis (up to 2 mm).

Counseling is an important part of laser treatment. Counseling should done regarding:
- Possibility of 20–30% chance of recommence
- Future risk of malignancy
- Importance of long-term follow-up as laser is an ablative procedure.

Advantages of laser therapy:
- Cosmetic value
- The procedure can be done in the outpatient setting
- The extent of tissue destruction can be controlled.

Disadvantages of laser therapy:
- Greater expertise is required
- It is a painful procedure
- Healing time is prolonged. 3 months required to heal the ulcer.
- No tissue can be obtained for histopathological examination.

Postoperative care after laser therapy:
- Routine analgesic and antibiotics should be prescribed to all cases for 7–10 days.
- Steroids are helpful given for 3–4 postoperative days.
- Vulvar folds should be kept apart for proper aeration, which will keep the lesion dry and help in healing the ulcer produced by laser therapy. Wound can be kept dry by the use of hair dryer.

- Sitz Bath should be given thrice a day for the clearance of the any infection.

Surveillance

Post-treatment recurrence rates exceed 30–50% with all treatment regimens and are higher with positive excision margins. In most studies, follow-up has been limited, and women with VIN should be considered to be at risk of recurrent VIN and vulvar cancer throughout their lifetimes. The value of vulvar self-examination and serial office visits in the detection of recurrence has not been proved prospectively, but both appear prudent. Given the relatively slow rate of progression, women with a complete response to therapy and no new lesions at follow-up visits scheduled 6 and 12 months after initial treatment should be monitored annually thereafter.

Regardless of treatment modality, recurrence of VIN is common. Even with modern treatment and management, invasive cancer will still develop in 3–5% of women, considerably higher than the risk of cervical cancer post-treatment of CIN. Recurrent VIN is a significant problem and represents both incomplete primary treatment and disease recurrence. Lifelong vigilance is an important component of the management of VIN.

Immune response modifiers: Surgery is the treatment of choice for VIN, but the surgical margins will be positive in 24–64% of cases. Surgery dose not eradicate HPV, the primary cause of VIN, which argues for the possible role of immune response modifiers in treatment.

Imiquimod (Aldara) is an imidazoquinoline, a novel synthetic compound that is a topical immune response stimulator. It enhances both innate and acquired immune pathways, particularly the T helper cell type I-mediated immune response, resulting in antiviral, anititumor, and immunoregulatory activities. HPV exclusively infects epithelial keratinocytes. The virus does not elicit cell death and infection is not accompanied by inflammation, which would normally activate the immune system. It is difficult for the host immune system to recognize the virus during the early stages of infection, which increases the risk for persistent infection.

Imiquimod alters the local immune response, which favors clearance of a persistent HPV infection.

HPV Vaccination

The very strong association between usual-type VIN and HPV 16 indicates that the current vaccination programs targeting HPV 16 and 18 should significantly impact future incidence of VIN and vulvar cancer. The FUTURE I and FUTURE II trials of the quadrivalent vaccine against HPVs 6, 11, 16 and 18 have demonstrated very high levels of protection against future development of usual-type VIN. This protection applied to the population of women who may have been already exposed to high-risk HPV types. Although the modal age of diagnosis of usual-type VIN has fallen substantially, current trials still exclude the age groups at greatest risk of this disease. As the majority of HPV-associated vulvar and vaginal cancers occur in the older age-groups, the ultimate benefits of vaccination are likely to take some years to be fully realized.

The use of vaccination against HPV 16 oncoproteins as a therapeutic strategy for women with usual-type VIN is very promising.

Prognosis

In younger patients spontaneous regression of VIN may occur. Untreated VIN has the potential of progression to invasive cancer. This risk may be as high as 100% for women over the age 40.

In surgically treated patients, women with pathological clear margins have a lower but still significant risk of recurrence compared with involved margins ACOG.

Gross margins of 0.5–1 cm around tissue with visible disease appear optimal, but decision of incision margin may be altered to avoid injury to the clitoris, urethra, anus or other critical structures.

Disaia reported a 39% recurrence rate in patients with VIN III treated by skinning vulvectomy with split-thickness skin grafting.

Conclusion

No treatment modality is ideal for every woman. Treatment should be individualized according to age, distribution, severity, associated disease, and previous treatment. Close follow-up after treatment remains essential because of the recurrent disease. Most recurrences occur within 3 years of treatment. Positive excision margin, multifocal disease, smoking, and immunosuppression are associated with increased recurrence rates.

PAGET'S DISEASE

Paget's disease of vulva is a nonsquamous intraepithelial neoplasia associated with proliferation of atypical glandular cells of apocrine type. It is sometimes associated with underlying invasive cancer.

Originally Paget's disease was described of a breast lesion (Sir James Paget, 1874) in which the appearance of the nipple heralded an underlying carcinoma. Extramammary Paget's disease account for 1–6% of all cases of Paget's disease. It predominantly affects women over 60 years of age and the vulva accounts for up to 60% of cases.

Classification

Recent classification of vulvar Paget's disease has been shown in Box 4.3. Grossly there are two types of extramammary Paget's disease. Types I Paget's disease is of primary cutaneous origin. Type II Paget's disease is of noncutaneous origin, such as the rectum, bladder or upper genital tract. Gynecological oncologists are concerned with type I cutaneous Paget's disease.

Clinical Features

The disease predominantly affects postmenopausal white women and presenting symptoms are usually pruritus and vulvar soreness. Microscopically the lesion has a deep red lesion surrounded by shiny

---

BOX 4.3: Classification of Paget's disease of the vulva.

1. Primary Paget's Disease of the Vulva
    a. Intraepithelial Paget's disease
    b. Intraepithelial Paget's disease with stromal invasion
    c. As a manifestation of an underlying adenocarcinoma of a skin appendage or subcutaneous vulvar gland
2. Secondary Paget's Disease of the Vulva
    a. Secondary to an anorectal adenocarcinoma
    b. Secondary to an urothelial carcinoma
    c. As a manifestation of another noncutaneous adenocarcinoma (e.g. endocervical, endometrial, ovarian)

Source: Modified from Berek JS Hacker NF. Berek and Hacker's Gynecologic Oncology, 6th edition. Philadelphia: Wolters Kluwer; 2014.

Vulvar Intraepithelial Neoplasia

white epithelium. The surface of the lesion is irregular. The lesion usually begins on the hair-bearing areas of the vulva. It may extend to involve the mons pubis, thighs and buttocks. Extension to involve the mucosa of the rectum vagina or urinary tract has also been described. The more extensive lesions are usually raised velvety in appearance and weep persistently (Figs. 4.5 and 4.6).

Microscopically, the epidermis contains large secretary cells arranged singly or in groups. These cells are called Paget's cell. The cells have abundant cytoplasm, which is pale and vacuolated, contain mucin, similar to that normally secreted by apocrine glands. The cell contains a large nucleus with a prominent nucleolus which is polymorphic and hyperchromatic. Most of the Paget's cells are in the basal layer of the epithelium (Figs. 4.7A to C).

Investigations

All patients should be screened for any associated malignancy. About 30–40% of Paget's disease are associated with adnexal carcinoma. Treatment of this group of patients is different. The investigations should include:
- Mammography
- Computed tomography (CT) scan of the pelvis and abdomen.

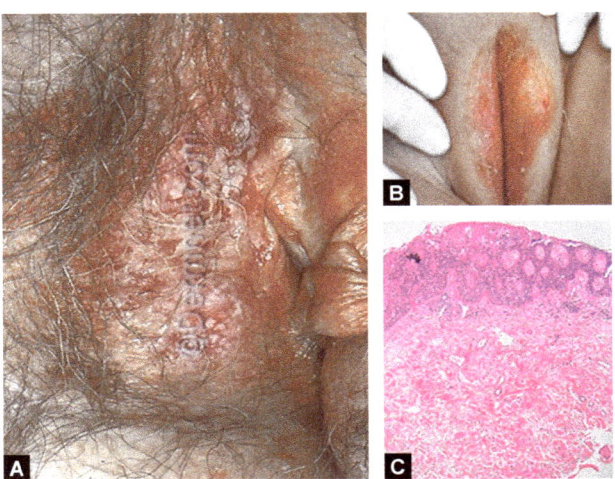

Figs. 4.5A to C: Paget's disease. (A) Hair-bearing areas of the vulva; (B) Extensive and weeping lesion of vulva. (C) Histological structure of the same.

60 Principles and Practices of Premalignant and Malignant Disorders of Vulva

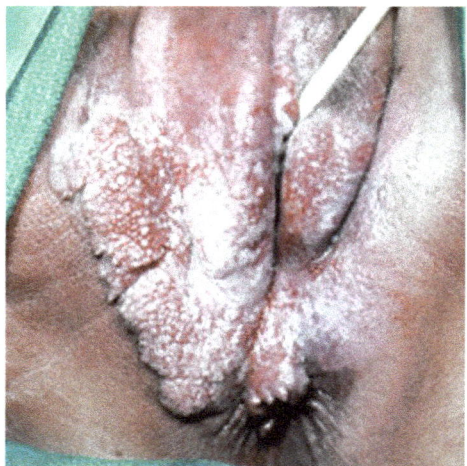

Fig. 4.6: Paget's disease of the labium majora.

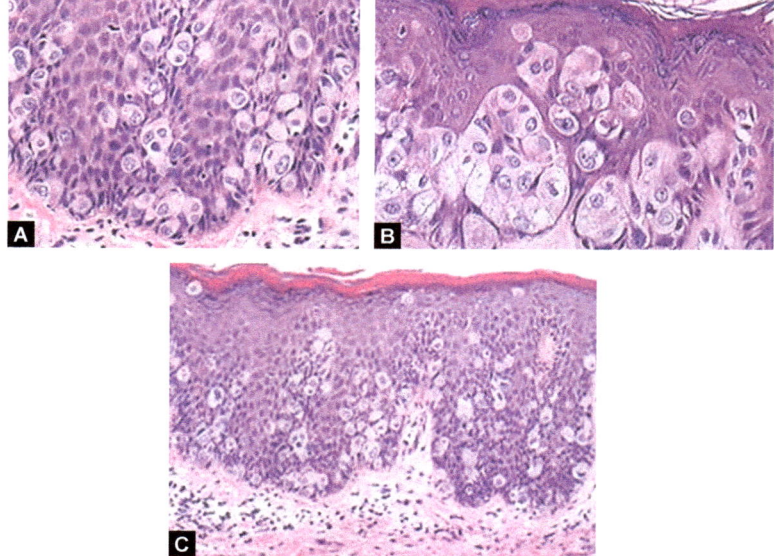

Figs. 4.7A to C: Histology of the Paget's disease. (A) The epidermis contains large secretary Paget's cells arranged singly or in groups. (B) The Paget's cells have abundant cytoplasm, which is pale and vacuolated and contain mucin. (C) Most of the Paget's cells are in the basal layer of the epithelium.
(*Source:* Clinical Gynecologic Pathology: Hernandez Atkinson; Diseases of the vulva; Cornelia Liu Trimble, Edward L. Trimble, J. Donald Woodruff: W.B Saunders Company, 1996, p.12)

- Transvaginal ultrasonography.
- Cervical cytology.
- Colonoscopy, if the disease involves the anus.
- Cystoscopy, if the disease involves the urethra.

Treatment

The mainstay of treatment is wide superficial resection of the gross disease. Underlying adenocarcinoma may or may not be clinically appearance. Paget's cell may invade the underlying dermis, which should be removed for adequate histological evaluation. That's why laser therapy is not satisfactory for primary Paget's disease. The surgical defect usually can be closed by primary closure or a split thickness skin graft may be required. Unlike squamous cell carcinoma in situ, in Paget's disease, the edge is ill-defined and the cells extend beyond the apparent clinical limits, resulting in frequent positive surgical margins. The group at Memorial Sloan-Kettering cancer center reported positive margins in 20–28 patients as 72%.

Surgical margins may be checked with frozen sections, these can be misleading and resection of the entire gross lesion with margins of at least 1 cm will control symptoms and exclude invasive disease.

There is a role of radiotherapy for vulvar Paget's disease when involves anus or urethra and surgery would involve diversion and stoma formation. Another alternative approach is to treat the lesion by photodynamic therapy. Recurrent lesions should be treated by further surgical resection. Topical imiquimod cream (5%) has been used successfully for recurrent Paget's disease.

Invasive Paget's Disease

When Paget's disease is associated with underlying invasive carcinoma, it should be treated in the same manner as a squamous vulvar cancer. These patients may require radical vulvectomy and at least an ipsilateral lymphadenectomy because lymph node metastases have been reported in patients with very superficially invasive Paget's disease. If lymph nodes are not dissected in a superficially invasive Paget's disease, the groin should be carefully monitored by ultrasound.

Prognosis

Paget's disease tends to recur locally over many years, not only due to multifocal distribution but also due to the fact that the edge is ill-defined and excision is often incomplete. Recurrent lesions are usually in situ. But 67% in British registry showed progression to invasive disease in 1 to 21 year after the initial diagnosis and treatment.

REFERENCES

1. Judson PL, Haberm B, Baxter NN, et al. Trends in the incidence of invasive and in situ vulvar carcinoma. Obstet Gynecol. 2006;107:1018-22.
2. De Vuyst H, Clifford GM, Nascimento MC, et al. Prevalence and type distribution of human papillomavirus in carcinoma and intraepithelial neoplasia of the vulva, vagina and anus: a meta-analysis. Int J Cancer. 2009;124(7):1626-36.
3. Sideri M, Jones RW, Wilkinson EJ, et al. Squamous vulvar intraepithelial neoplasia: 2004 modified terminology, ISSVD Vulvar Oncology Subcommittee. J Reprod Med. 2005;50:807-10.
4. Sturgeon SR, Curtis RF, Johnson K, et al. Second primary cancers after vulvar and vaginal cancers. Am J Obstet Gynecol. 1996;174:929-33.
5. Eva LJ, Ganesan R, Chan KK, et al. Differentiated-type vulval intraepithelial neoplasia has a high-risk association with vulval squamous cell carcinoma. Int J Gynecol Cancer. 2009;19:741-4.
6. Van da Nieuwenhof HP, Massuger LF, van der Avort IA, et al. Vulvar squamous cell carcinoma development after diagnosis of VIN increases with age. Eur J Cancer. 2009;45:851-6.
7. Rodke G, Friedrich EG Jr, Wilkinson EJ. Malignant potential of mixed vulvar dystrophy (lichen associated with squamous cell hyperplasia). J Reprod Med. 1988;33:545-50.
8. Carli P, De Magnis A, Mannone F, et al. Vulvar carcinoma associated with lichen sclerosus. Experience at the Florence, Italy. Vulvar Clinic J Reprod Med. 2003;48:313-8.
9. Scurry J. Does lichen sclerosus play a central role in the pathogenesis of human papillomavirus negative squamous cell carcinoma? The itch-scrath-licerosus hypothesis. Int J Gynaecol Cancer.1999;89-97.
10. Sideri M, Jones RW, Wilkinson EJ, et al. Squamous vulvar intraepithelial neoplasia: 2004 modified terminology, ISSVD Vulvar Oncology Subcommittee. J Reprod Med. 2005;50:807-10.
11. Shylasree TS, Karanjgaokar V, Tritram A, et al. Contribution of dermographic, psychological and disease-related factors to quality of

life in women with high-grade vulval intraepithelial neoplasia. Gynecol Oncol. 2008;110(2):185-9.
12. Jones RW, Rowan DM. Spontaneous regression of vulvar intraepithelial neoplasia 2-3. Obstet Gynecol. 2000.96(3):470-2.
13. Van Seters M, van beurden M, ten Kate FJ, et al. Treatment of vulvar intraepithelial neoplasia with topical imiquimod: seven years median follow-up of a randomized clinical trial. N Engl J Med. 2008;358:1465-73.
14. Sideri M, Spinaci L, Spolti N, et al. Evaluation of CO_2 laser excision or vaporization for the treatment of vulvar intraepithelial neoplasia. Gynecol Oncol. 1999;75:277-81.
15. Reid R. Superficial laser vulvectomy. III. A new surgical technique for appendage-conserving ablation of refractory condylomas and vulvar intraepithelial neoplasia. Am J Obstet Gynecol. 1985;152:504-9.

CHAPTER 5

Vulvar Cancer (Squamous Type)

INTRODUCTION

Vulvar cancer is uncommon, representing approximately 4% of all female genital cancers. 80% of vulvar cancers are squamous cell type. The incidence of in situ vulvar cancer has been more than doubled over the past two decades, whereas the rate of invasive squamous cell carcinoma of vulva has remained stable.

COMPOSITION OF VULVA

The vulva is a composite structure consisting of the mons pubis, labia majora, labia minora, clitoris and mucosa of the lower third of the vagina and urethra. Vulvar cancer arises from skin, subcutaneous tissue, sweat glands, sebaceous glands, Bartholin's glands, and mucosa of the lower third of the vagina.

CLASSIFICATION OF VULVAR CANCER ACCORDING TO HISTOPATHOLOGY

Two main subdivisions of vulvar cancer on the basis of histopathology are:

Squamous Cell Type

- Squamous cell carcinoma (Epidermoid Cancer)
- Verrucous carcinoma.

Nonsquamous Cell Type

- Malignant melanoma
- Adenocarcinoma of Bartholin's gland
- Basal cell carcinoma
- Extramammary Paget's disease with underlying adenocarcinoma
- Sarcoma
- Lymphoma
- Endodermal sinus tumor
- Secondary metastatic tumor.

INCIDENCE AND EPIDEMIOLOGY

Only 5% of gynecological cancers and 0.6% of all female cancers arises from vulvar cancer.[1] In 2014, an estimated 4,850 new cases of vulvar cancer were diagnosed and there was 1,030 deaths in United States. Squamous cell carcinomas account for 85–90% of cases, were basal cell carcinomas, invasive Paget's disease, Bartholin gland carcinomas, and sarcomas are much less common. It is common in low socioeconomic and elderly women. No race, culture and color are immune to vulvar cancer. It is the disease of postmenopausal women, with increasing age the incidence of vulvar cancer increases. So it is common in the 7th and 8th decade of life. Peak age group is between 60 years and 70 years. Average age of diagnosis is 65 years. But 75% patients are more than 50 years of age and 15% patients are less than 40 years of age.

ETIOLOGY

Etiological factors in young and older women are different. Human papillomavirus (HPV) infection is strongly associated with vulvar cancer in younger women.[2,3] Often it is associated with VIN and CIN. About 20–60% of patients are found to be HPV DNA positive, and about 85% of HPV positive invasive vulvar cancers are attributable to high risk HPV 16. In 22% cases of vulvar cancer CIN or invasive cancer cervix has been reported.

In older women, invasive vulvar cancer frequently is preceded by vulvar intraepithelial neoplasia (VIN). Squamous cell hyperplasia type of vulvar dystrophy is a predisposing or associated condition of squamous cell type of vulvar cancer in older women. Chronic pruritus is an important antecedent factor.

Tobacco smoking and multiple sexual partners are important cofactors. There has been a significant increase in the incidence of VIN in recent decades[4-7] and this has been attributed to changing sexual behavior, HPV infection, and cigarette smoking.[8]

DIAGNOSTIC DILEMMAS

Vulvar cancer is predominantly a disease of older women. In spite of the vulva being an external organ, delayed diagnosis has been typical of this disease. It is a slowly growing, well differentiated surface tumor and expected to be diagnosed early. The causes for the cases not being diagnosed early have been identified as:
- There is delay in reporting to the doctors by 6–12 months
- 25% of the patients consult a physician for pruritus without having a biopsy
- Tendency of the consultants for taking incomplete excisional biopsy may miss the proper diagnosis.

Suspicious Points for Early Diagnosis of Vulvar Cancer

Some associated conditions may raise the suspicion of vulvar cancer. Associated conditions are:
- Obesity creates an environment of warmth and moisture of the vulva which favors both HPV and other infections to produce intense inching and some epithelial changes of vulva.
- *Hypertension:* 30–50% of squamous cell type vulvar cancer patients are obese and hypertensive.
- *Diabetes:* 10% patients are diabetic. Diabetes causes chronic vulvar irritation and pruritus which may act as antecedent factors of squamous type vulvar cancer.
- Sexually transmitted diseases like lymphogranuloma venereum, granuloma inguinale and syphilis, may be associated with vulvar cancer.
- Squamous cell hyperplasia type of vulvar dystrophy or lichen sclerosis may be associated with squamous cell type of invasive vulvar cancer.

- In younger women, CIN, VIN, and VAIN may be associated with invasive type of vulvar cancer.

TYPES OF SQUAMOUS CELL CARCINOMA OF VULVA

Squamous cell type carcinoma of vulva arises from the anterior half of the vulva. 65% of this cancer arises from labia majora and minora and 25% arises from the clitoris and perineum. 33% of cases are bilateral or midline in position. Macroscopically four types of carcinomas are found:
1. *Exophytic cauliflower-like lesion:* This type of lesion starts with malodorous necrotic growth, and presents as a large lesion (Figs. 5.1 to 5.4).
2. *Ulcerative type (ulcer crater):* The lesion starts with raised, flat, white, hypertrophic lump. Later on the lump undergoes traumatized breaking down its surface to give rise to a small ulcer crater. The ulcer gradually increases in size involving the surrounding tissue (Fig. 5.5).
3. Slightly elevated, reddish velvety tumors, which gradually spread over the skin surface.
4. *Verrucous type lesion:* These are hyperkeratotic papilla, multiple in number, histologically papillary growths without a central core of connective tissue.

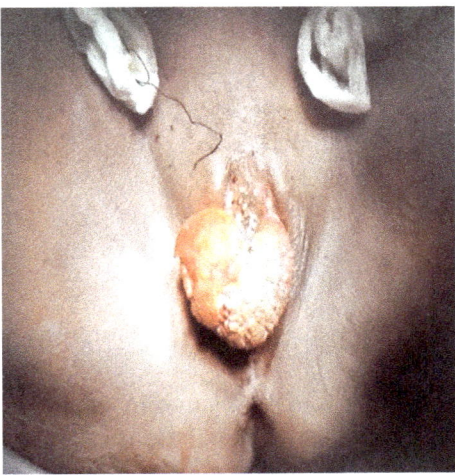

Fig. 5.1: Exophytic growth over vulva and clitoris.

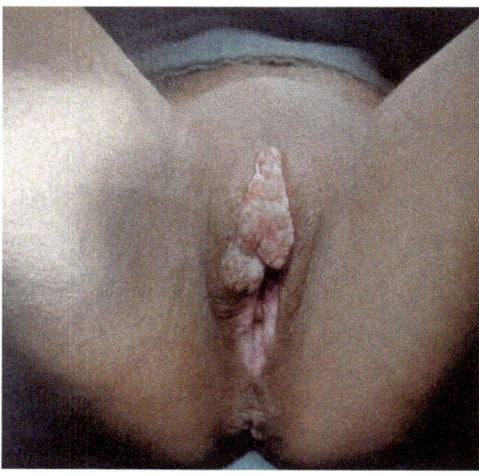

Fig. 5.2: Squamous carcinoma of vulva arising from clitoris extending over right labia majora with leukoplakia.

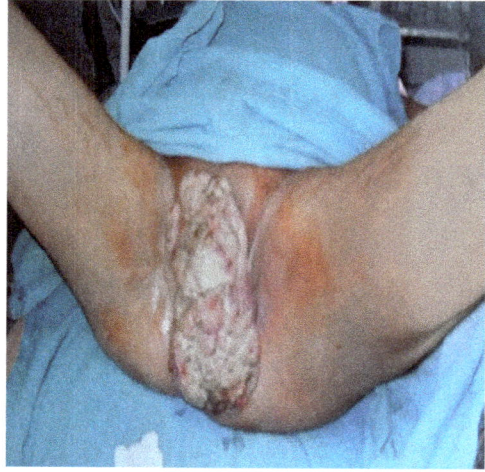

Fig. 5.3: A large exophytic growth covering whole vulva and perineum.

The gross appearances of the lesions do not give any clues about grading, prognosis or metastasis. It is the gross size of the tumor which is the most significant factor in prognosis of the carcinoma.

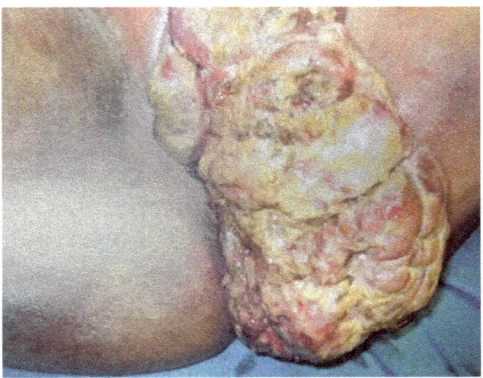

Fig. 5.4: A large exophytic growth with surface ulceration and foul smell discharge.

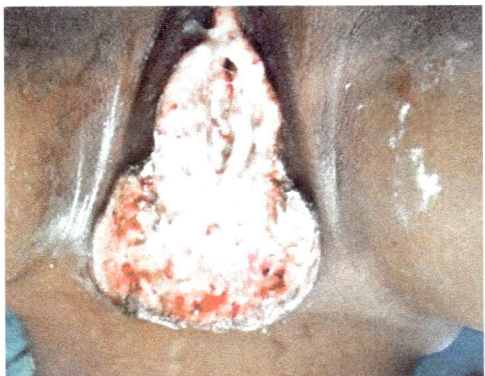

Fig. 5.5: Whole of vulva eaten by the growth resulting in big ulcer.
[*Source:* Dr Jitendra Pariyar, Fellowship in Gynecologic Oncology, Junior Consultant, BP Koirala Memorial Cancer Hospital, Chitwan, Nepal (Figs. 5.1 to 5.5).]

Clinical Profile of Squamous Vulvar Cancer

These patients present with some common general criteria.
- 30–50% patients are obese and hypertensive
- 10% are diabetic
- It is a disease of 7th and 8th decade of life
- Only 15% patients are of less than 40 years of age
- 20% of patients have a secondary primary carcinoma, 75% of them in the cervix

- Other sites of second primary carcinoma are kidney, urethra, breast and Bartholin's gland.

Clinical Presentations of Squamous Vulvar Cancer

- Earliest symptom of vulvar cancer is pruritus. Later on mass develop, 50% of the patients develop or lump. Most patients present with a vulvar lump or mass, although there is open a long history of pruritus, usually associated with a vulvar dystrophy.
- The less common presentations are dominated by local pain, bleeding and surface drainage from the tumors and ulcerations. In advanced stage there may be large metastatic mass together with these presentations.
- In 20% cases are incidental findings with no complaints.
- 25% patients give history of consultation with physician without the benefit of biopsy.
- In some cases, an incomplete biopsy without final diagnosis shifts the dilemma of diagnosis.

Physical Examination Findings

On physical examination, the lesion is usually raised and may be fleshy, ulcerated, leukoplakic, or warty in appearance. Warty lesions are often initially misdiagnosed as condylomata acuminate.

Most squamous carcinomas of the vulva occur on the labia majora, but the labia minora, clitoris, and perineum also may be primary sites. A study from one University Hospital in Germany reported a recent change in location of the tumor, with 37% of occurring between the clitoris and urethra in the 10 years up to 2007, compared to 19% in the 1980s ($p < 0.050$). Approximately 10% of the cases are too extensive to determine a site of origin, and approximately 5% of the cases are multifocal.

As part of the clinical assessment, the growth lymph nodes should be palpated, a Papanicolaou smear taken from the cervix, and colposcopy of the cervix and vagina performed because of the common association with other squamous intraepithelial neoplasms of the lower genital tract.

Diagnostic Evaluation

Initial evaluation should include a detailed analysis of the patient's history and a thorough physical and gynecological examination. Special emphasis should be given to identify the following factors:
- Measurements of the primary tumor
- Assessment of extension to adjacent mucosal or body structures
- Possible involvement of the inguinal lymph nodes
- Because neoplasia of the female genital tract is often multifocal, evaluation of the cervix and vagina by cytologic screening test should always be performed.
- Fine needle aspiration cytology from sites of suspected metastasis may eliminate the need for surgical exploration in some patients with advanced tumors.

Diagnosis of many cases of vulvar cancer is simple and easy, provided clinical features of the patient are thoroughly evaluated. Optimal diagnosis for any patient presenting with a suspicious lesion is to proceed directly to biopsy under local anesthesia. Tissue biopsies should include the cutaneous lesions in question and contagious underlying stoma so that the presence of invasion and depth of invasion can be accurately assessed. The goals of immediate evaluation with outpatient biopsy are to avoid delay in the planning of appropriate therapy. It is preferable to leave the primary lesion in situ to allow the treating surgeon to fashion adequate surgical margins.

Differential Diagnosis

- Vulvar dystrophy
- Vulvar diffuse white lesions or leukoplakia
- Vulvar ulcerative lesions, like syphilitic ulcer, herpetic ulcer, tubercular ulcer
- Discrete benign tumors of the vulva.

Routes of Spread

Vulvar cancers metastasize in three ways:
1. Local growth and extension into adjacent organs such as the urethra, vagina and away.
2. Lymphatic embolism or permeation to regional lymph nodes in the groin.

3. Hematogenous dissemination to distant sites, including the lungs, liver and bone.[1]

Hematogenous spread usually occurs late in the course of vulva cancer and is rare in the absence of lymph node metastases. Hematogenous spread is uncommon in patients with one or two positive groin nodes, but is more common in patients with three or more positive nodes.

Descriptions of local extension are clinically useful in that the local surgical resection with a wide margin is almost universally feasible in women with T1 and T2 tumors, occasionally possible in T3 lesions and almost impossible in T4 tumors.

Most recent experience with intraoperative mapping has demonstrated that lymphatic drainage from most vulvar sites proceeds initially to a "sentinel" node located within the superficial inguinal group of lymph nodes.

STAGING SYSTEM[2]

International Federation of Gynecology and Obstetrics (FIGO) adopted a modified surgical staging system in 1989, which remained relatively unchanged in their 1995 recommendations.

A new FIGO Staging System for Vulvar Cancer was introduced in 2009 (Table 5.1), to address the above issues. Stage IA remains unchanged, but Stages I and II have been combined. The 2009 staging system shifted patients who have distal vaginal, distal urethral or anal involvement from the T3 to the T2 category and if lymph nodes are negative then FIGO stage III is shifted to FIGO stage II. This shift classifies patients more accurately according to prognosis, which is dominated by the nodal status but the new T2 category includes patients who are treated with surgery alone, together with lesions that may be treated with initial radiation to preserve urethral or anal function.

PREDICTING LYMPH NODE METASTASIS

Lymphatic metastases may occur early in the disease. Initially, spread is usually to the inguinal lymph nodes, which are located between Camper's fascia and the fascia lata. From these superficial groin

TABLE 5.1: International Federation of Gynecology and Obstetrics (FIGO) surgical staging for vulvar cancer (2009).

FIGO stage	TNM	Clinical/Pathologic findings
Stage I		Tumor confined to the vulva
IA	T1a, N0, M0	Lesions ≤2 cm in size, confined to the vulva or perineum and with stromal invasion ≤ 1.0 mm*, no nodal metastasis.
IB	T1b, N0, M0	Lesion >2 cm in size or with stromal invasion >1.0 mm*, confined to the vulva or perineum, no nodal metastasis.
Stage II	T2, N0, M0	Tumor of any size with extension to adjacent perineal structures (one-third lower urethra, one-third lower vagina, anus) with negative nodes.
Stage III		Tumor of any size with or without extension to adjacent perineal structures (one-third lower urethra, one-third lower vagina, anus) with positive inguinofemoral lymph nodes.
IIIA	T1, T2, N1a, M0 T1, T2, N1b, M0	i. 1–2 lymph node metastasis (<5 mm), or ii. 1 lymph node metastasis (es) (≥ 5 mm).
IIIB	T1, T2, N2a, M0 T1, T2, N2b, M0	i. ≥3 lymph node metastasis (<5 mm), or ii. ≥2 lymph node metastasis (es) (≥ 5 mm).
IIIC	T1, T2, N2c, M0	With positive nodes with extracapsular spread.
Stage IV		Tumor invades other regional (two-thirds upper urethra, two-thirds upper vagina), or distant structures.
IVA	T1, T2, T3, N3, M0	Tumor invades any of the following: i. Upper urethral and/or vaginal mucosa, bladder mucosa, rectal mucosa, or fixed to pelvic bone, or ii. Fixed or ulcerated inguinofemoral lymph nodes.
IVB	Any T, any N, M1	Any distant metastasis including pelvic lymph nodes.

*The depth of invasion is defined as the measurement of the tumor from the epithelial–stromal junction of the adjacent most superficial dermal papilla to the deepest point of invasion.

nodes, the disease spreads to the femoral nodes, which are located medial to the femoral vein. Cloquet's node, situated beneath the inguinal ligament, is the most cephalad of the femoral node group. Metastases to the femoral nodes without involvement of the inguinal nodes have reported.

From the inguinofemoral nodes, the cancer spreads to the pelvic nodes, particularly the external iliac group. Although direct lymphatic pathways from the clitoris and Bartholin gland to the pelvic nodes have been described, these channels seem to be of minimal clinical significance.

Since 1980s, the overall incidence of lymph node metastases is reported to be approximately 30%. The incidence of lymph node metastasis in relation to clinical stage of the disease is shown in Table 5.2.

Metastases to pelvic nodes are uncommon, the overall reported frequency being approximately 9%. About 20% of patients with positive groin nodes have positive pelvic nodes. Pelvic nodal metastases are rare in the absence of clinically suspicious (N2) groin nodes, three or more positive groin nodes and a tumor with invasion more than 4 mm.

The presence of certain parameters can be taken as a predictor for lymph node metastasis.
- Lesion size is greater than 2 cm
- Poorly differentiated tumor
- Increasing depth of stromal invasion
- Lymphovascular space involvement present in initial biopsy specimen.

TABLE 5.2: Incidence of lymph node metastases in relation to clinical stage disease.

Stage	No. of cases	Positive nodes	Percent
I	140	15	10.7
II	145	38	26.2
III	137	88	64.2
IV	18	16	88.9

Source: Data compiled from Green, 1978; Lversen et al., 1980; and Hacker et al., 1983.

Clinically Important Observations Regarding Nodal Metastasis

The superficial inguinal nodes are the most frequent site of metastasis. Nodal involvement proceeds in stepwise fashion from superficial inguinal nodes to the deep inguinal nodes and then to the external iliac group of nodes.

- In transit metastases within the vulvar skin are exceedingly rare, suggesting that most initial lymphatic metastases represent an embolic phenomenon
- Contralateral lymph node spread is common as a result of the intercommunicating lymphatic system between the two sides of the vulvar skin
- Contralateral lymph node metastasis is unusual in the absence of ipsilateral groin node metastasis
- Spread to the pelvic lymph nodes is considered to be distant metastasis. It is found in only 3% of cases, where the growth is midline or central in position and bilateral in distribution.

TREATMENT

After the pioneering work of Taussig[3] in the United States and Way[4,5] in Great Britain, en bloc radical vulvectomy and bilateral dissection of the groin and pelvic nodes became the standard treatment for most patients with operable vulvar cancer. If the disease involved the anus, rectovaginal septum, or proximal urethra, some type of pelvic exenteration was combined with this dissection.

Although the survival rate improved markedly with this aggressive surgical approach, several factors have led to modifications of this "standard" treatment plan during the past 25 years. These factors include earlier presentation of affected women in Western countries, and increasing concern among patients and doctors about the physical and psychosexual morbidity associated with radical vulvectomy.

Modern management of vulvar cancer requires an experienced, multidisciplinary team approach, which is available only in tertiary referral centers. Successful centralization of the management of patients with vulvar cancer occurred in the eastern part of the Netherlands following the release of national guidelines by the Dutch

Society of Obstetrics and Gynecology in 2000. As the incident of this disease is very low and its treatment requires a highly specialized technique, centralization management of these patients is essential.

Management of Early Stage Vulvar Cancers

The modern approach to the management of patients with carcinoma confined to the vulva should be individualized.[6] There is no "standard" treatment applicable to every patient, and emphasis is given to performing the most conservative operative procedure which will be most suitable for the cure of the disease.

In considering the appropriate operation, it is necessary to determine the appropriate management of following:
1. The primary lesion
2. The groin lymph nodes.

Before any surgery, every patient should have colposcopy of the cervix, vagina and vulva, because preinvasive (and rarely invasive) lesions may be present at other sites in addition to the lower genital tract.

Management of the Primary Lesion—the two factors which should be taken into account when determining the management of the primary tumor are the following:
- The condition of the remainder of the vulva
- The presence or absence of multifocal invasive disease

Although radical vulvectomy has been regarded as the standard treatment for the primary malignant vulvar lesion, this operation is associated with significant disturbances of sexual function and body image. Andersen and Hacker[7] reported that, when compared with healthy adult women, sexual arousal was reduced to the eighth percentile and body image to the fourth percentile in women who had undergone radical vulvectomy.

Since the early 1980s, several investigators have advocated a radical local excision rather than a radical vulvectomy for the primary lesion in patients with T1 and T2 tumors.[8] Regardless of whether a radical vulvectomy or a radical local excision is performed, surgical margins will be the same and an analysis of the available literature indicates that the incidence of local invasive recurrence is low if the histopathologic margin (after fixation) is at least 8 mm.[9] Allowing for

20% tissue shrinkage with formalin, surgical free margin should be at least 1 cm.

When vulvar cancer arises in the presence of VIN or some non-neoplastic disorder, radical local excision should be performed for the invasive disease and the associated disease should be treated in the most appropriate manner.

For example, topical steroids may be required for squamous hyperplasia or lichen sclerosus, whereas VIN should be treated by superficial local excision and primary closure or split thickness skin grafting.

Radical local excision of the invasive lesion is most appropriate for lesions on the lateral or posterior aspect of the vulva where preservation of the clitoris is feasible. For patients with anterior lesions, surgical resections that include clitorectomy can have serious psychosexual consequences, particularly in younger patients.

In young patients with actual involvement of the clitoris or for whom surgical margins would be less than 5 mm, consideration should be given to treating the primary lesion with a small field of radiation therapy. Small vulvar lesions can often be controlled with 62–64 Gy of external radiation. If there is suspicion of persistent diseases, biopsy can be performed after therapy to confirm complete response.[10]

Operative Treatment

Preoperative Investigations

These patients are usually elderly with malnutrition and some medical comorbidities. Often these patients present with some undiagnosed medical comorbidities and require diagnosis and management of these comorbidities prior to the operative procedure for vulvar cancer. Investigations should be individualized according to the examination findings. The investigations required for the purpose of treatment of these patients are:

- *Colposcopy of cervix:* Vulvar carcinoma may be associated with cervical cancer as both are caused by the HPV virus. Exclusion of cervical preinvasive or invasive disease is mandatory. This can be ensured by a Pap smear for cervical preinvasive disease followed by colposcopy and directed biopsy.

- *Colposcopy of vulva*: Sometimes the lesion is too small to identify. Knowing the extension of the disease is important for staging. Colposcopy directed biopsy is helpful in this regard.
- Examination under anesthesia (EUA) and endometrial biopsy should be performed if patient's complaint is irregular per vaginal bleeding, or postmenopausal bleeding.
- Other routine tests for evaluation of the patient's general condition are a complete blood count, routine urine test with or without culture and sensitivity test, blood sugar: fasting and two hours after 75 g of glucose, serum creatinine, serum SGPT, serum FT4 and TSH, HBSAg, ECG and chest X-ray.
- Special investigations are—proctoscopy/sigmoidoscopy according to rectal examination findings, intravenous pyelography according to ultrasonography (USG) findings, and Barium follow through if there is suggestive clinical feature of intestinal involvement.
- Computed tomography (CT) scanning of the whole abdomen should be done when an abdominal mass is identified by abdominal examination.
- Magnetic resonance imaging (MRI) can assist evaluation of the disease stage, especially in the case of advanced stage disease.

Preoperative Preparation

- Counseling is an essential step before surgery because extensive surgery may be necessary and may result in difficult complications, like disfiguration, dysuria, dyspareunia, urinary incontinence and difficulty in walking. Counseling should be thorough, including detailed information regarding extensiveness of surgery, probable perioperative and postoperative complications, cost of operation, and postoperative adjuvant therapy.
- Mechanical bowel preparation should be done in the usual way if anus and rectum are involved.
- Two units of whole blood should be kept ready to combat any perioperative or postoperative excessive bleeding.

Surgical Procedure

Primary treatment of vulvar cancer is complete surgical removal of all tumors. Staging and treatment of vulvar cancer are surgical.

The development of radical vulvectomy with bilateral inguino-femoral lymphadenectomy during the 1940s and 1950s was a dramatic improvement over prior surgical options and greatly enhanced survival, particularly with smaller tumors and negative nodes. Long-term survival of 85–90% can now be routinely obtained with radical surgery. However radical surgery can be associated with postoperative complications such as disfiguration, wound breakdown, and lymphedema. More recently emphasis has been given to individualize the tumor at either end of the spectrum.

Many gynecologists believe that smaller vulvar tumors can be acceptably managed by less radical surgical approaches. Advantages of such an approach are as follows:
- Retention of significant portion of uninvolved vulva
- Less operative morbidity
- Fewer late complications
- Radical surgery is frequently ineffective in curing patients with bulky tumors and positive groin nodes.

So, most commonly done surgery is wide radical local excision of the primary tumor with superficial and deep inguinal node dissection.

Management of Primary Lesion

Microinvasive tumor: Tumors demonstrating early invasion of the vulvar stroma (≤ 1 mm) have minimal risk for lymphatic dissemination. Excisional procedures that incorporate a 1 cm normal tissue margin are likely to provide a curative result. For this group of patients, evaluation of groin lymph nodes is unnecessary. After primary therapy, these patients should undergo frequent follow-up examination. No adjuvant radiotherapy is needed.

Stage I and II disease: In an effort to reduce morbidity and enhance psychosexual recovery, a more limited surgical approach has been employed by several groups of researchers. The most frequent recommendation is to resect the primary lesion with a 1–2 cm margin of normal tissue and to carry the dissection to the deep perineal fascia up to the interior fascia of urogenital diaphragm. This partial radical vulvectomy should not be confused with the concept of excisional biopsy, which is used primarily as a diagnostic procedure. In an attempt to reduce the treatment related morbidity, the classic radical operation has been replaced by the use of "triple incision" technique, i.e. separate vulvectomy and two groin incisions (Figs. 5.6 to 5.9).

Technique for radical local excision: Radical local excision implies a wide and deep excision of primary tumor. An elliptical incision should be drawn using a marking pen, with the skin in its natural position. Surgical margins around the tumor should be at least 1 cm away from

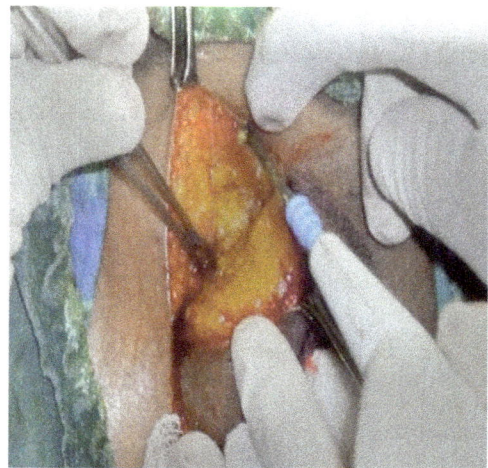

Fig. 5.6: Simple vulvectomy started by oval incision.

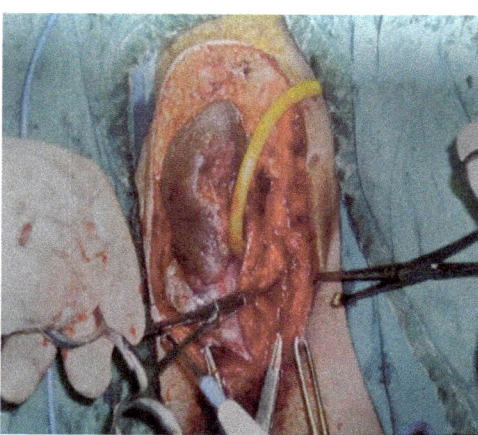

Fig. 5.7: Simple vulvectomy procedure.

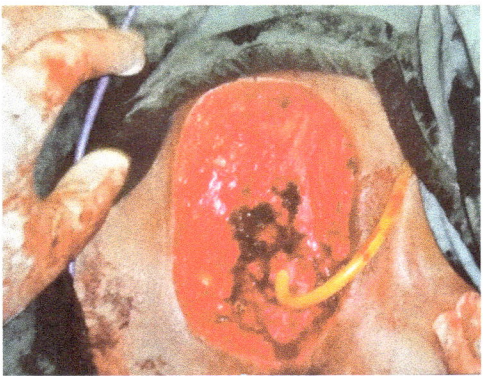

Fig. 5.8: Simple vulvectomy—specimen removed and catheter in situ.

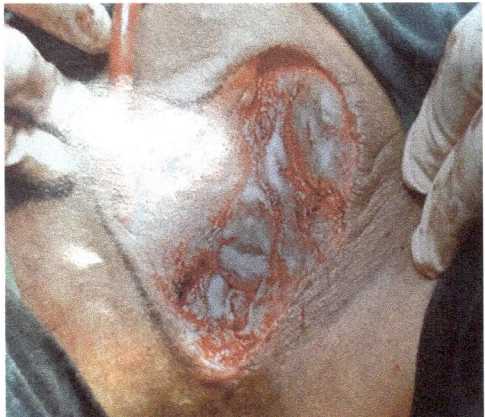

Fig. 5.9: Post simple vulvectomy drain tube in situ.

the tumor margin. The incision should be carried down to the inferior fascia of urogenital diaphragm, which is coplanar with the fascia lata and the fascia over the pubic symphysis. The surgical defect is closed in two layers. For perianal lesions, proximity to the anus may preclude adequate surgical margin, and in such cases consideration should be given to preoperative radiation. For periurethral lesions, the distal half of the urethra may be resected without loss of continence. Figures 5.10 and 5.11 show the satisfactory cosmetic result achieved in the treatment of the lesion.

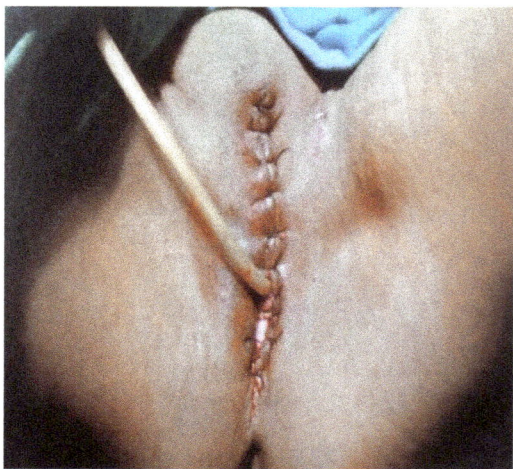

Fig. 5.10: Post simple vulvectomy and closer of the wound.

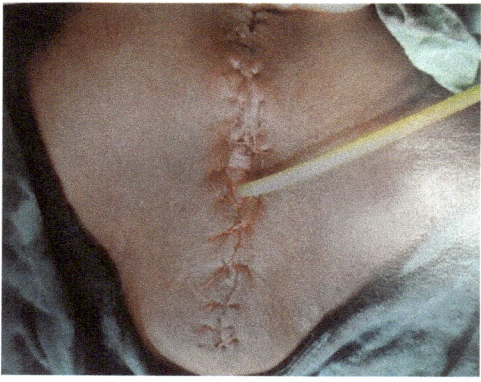

Fig. 5.11: Post simple vulvectomy and primary closer of the wound.

Management of the Groin Lymph Nodes

Appropriate management of the regional lymph nodes is the single most important factor in decreasing the mortality from early vulvar cancer. Most preoperative diagnostic dilemmas related to enlarged groin nodes can be resolved simply and accurately by using fine needle aspiration biopsy. Selective excision of groin lymph nodes may be considered when fine needle aspiration biopsy results are negative or equivocal, or to remove bulky positive nodes before beginning a course of combined modality therapy.

Inguinofemoral lymphadenectomy: It involves the removal of the lymph nodes in the groin. The femoral lymph nodes lie medial to the femoral vein beneath the cribriform fascia. This space contains the channel of lymph nodes which courses beneath the inguinal ligament and continues in the pelvis as the external iliac nodal chain. The most superior inguinal node is known as Cloquet node. In most cases, the surgical removal of the inguinofemoral lymph nodes is performed through separate groin incisions.

Technique for groin dissection: A linear incision is made 1 cm above and parallel to the groin crease along the medial three quarters of a line drawn between the anterior superior iliac spine and labiocrural fold (Fig. 5.12). This incision will be directly over the fossa ovalis (Fig. 5.12). Studies of bipedal lymphangiograms have demonstrated that there are no lymph nodes adjacent to the anterior superior iliac spine.[11] On the basis of embryologic and anatomical studies, Micheletti et al.[12] have proposed that the superficial circumflex iliac vessel could represent the lateral surgical landmark. The incision is carried through the subcutaneous tissues to the superficial Camper's fascia. This layer can be definitively identified, because the superficial circumflex iliac and superficial external pudendal vein runs immediately below it. The superficial fascia is incised and grasped with artery forceps to place it

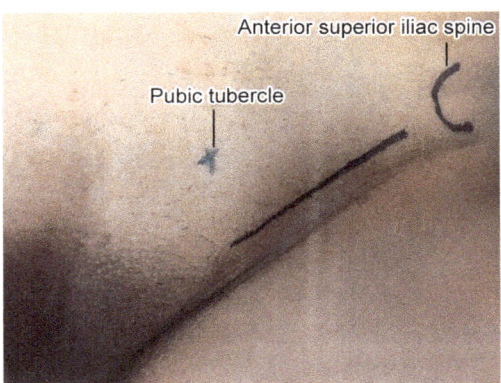

Fig. 5.12: Surgical marking for groin dissection.

on traction, and the fatty tissue between it and the fascia lata is removed over the femoral triangle (Figs. 5.13 and 5.14). To avoid skin necrosis, all subcutaneous tissue above the Camper fascia must be preserved. The dissection is carried up to 1 cm above the inguinal ligament to include all the inguinal nodes. The saphenous vein is usually tied off at the apex of the femoral triangle at its point in to the femoral vein.

The fatty tissue containing the femoral lymph nodes is removed from within the fossa ovalis. There are only one to three femoral

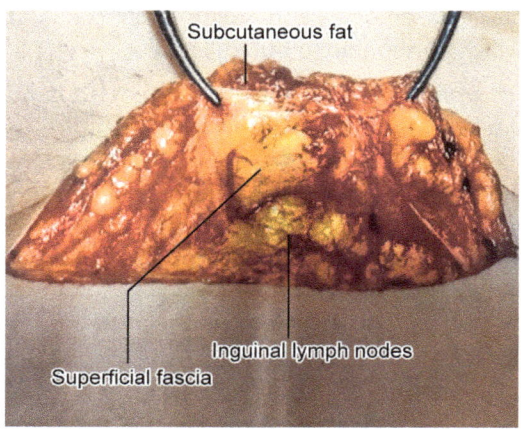

Fig. 5.13: Femoral triangle showing superficial fascia, inguinal lymph node and subcutaneous fat.

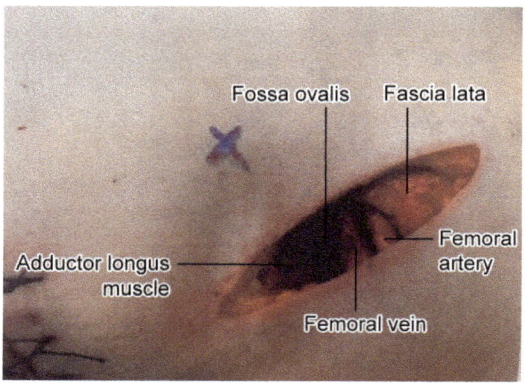

Fig. 5.14: Groin incision is directly over the fossa ovalis.
(Source: Berek JS, Hacker NF. Berek & Hacker's Gynecologic Oncology, 6th edition. Philadelphia: Wolters Kluwer; 2014)

lymph nodes, and they are always situated medial to the femoral vein in the opening of the fossa ovalis.[13] Hence, there is no need to remove the fascia lata lateral to the femoral vessels. Cloquet's node is not consistently present but should be investigated by retraction of the inguinal ligament cephalad over the femoral canal. The wound is closed in two layers, tacking the superficial fascia to the deep fascia. Placement of a drain in the groin is optional.

Indications of ipsilateral groin node dissection:
- Deep stromal involvement is > 1 mm.
- Lesion is at least 1 cm lateral to midline.
- Lesion is unilateral and >2 cm away from midline.

Indications of bilateral inguinofemoral (groin) node dissection:
- Lesion is bilateral.
- Lesion is central in position, i.e. within 2 cm of midline.
- Lesion encroaches on midline structures, i.e. clitoris, urethra or perineal body.

Superficial nodes are first removed and sent for frozen section biopsy. In patients with negative inguinal nodes, no further dissection or postoperative therapy is required.

Patients with positive nodes can undergo additional nodal dissection of contralateral groin or by irradiation or both. Patients with lymphadenectomy followed by irradiation have the greatest likelihood of development of lymphedema.

Lymphatic mapping: The major morbidity associated with the modern management of vulvar cancer is chronic lower limb lymphedema, which occurs in 60% patients following groin dissection, and is a lifelong affliction. Hence for the last 30 years, there has been much interest in eliminating or modifying the groin dissection for patients with negative nodes. Another surgical concept under evaluation is the potential for cutaneous lymphatic mapping to define and target the true sentinel groin nodes (Fig. 5.15). Preliminary experience with both intraoperative lymphatic dye and radioisotope injections suggest that a sentinel node can often be identified in the groin. By this method, lymphatic metastasis assessment can often be accomplished through biopsy of 1–2 identifiable nodes. If this concept proves sensitive and specific, more extensive inguinal lymphadenectomy might be abandoned.

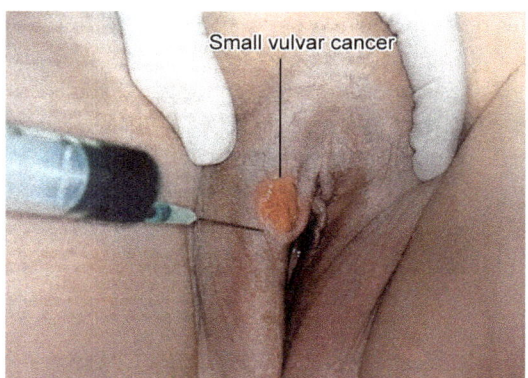

Fig. 5.15: Lymphatic mapping: injection of dye.

The concept of a "sentinel lymph node" suggests that the sentinel lymph node is the first lymph node in the lymphatic pathway and the primary site of metastasis.

There are two procedures for sentinel lymph node identification.
1. Use of an intraoperative blue dye staining technique.
2. Lymphoscintigraphy using radioactive 99mTc administered shortly before surgery, combined with intraoperative use of a hand held gamma probe.

Using both the methods in a patient during the operation produces the highest sensitivity of sentinel lymph node identification. Advantage of sentinel lymph node biopsy is that, as sentinel lymph nodes are subjected to a more rigorous pathologic examination, it permits the detection of smaller tumor foci compared to complete groin node dissection and traditional pathologic examination.

Factors for failure of sentinel lymph node identification:
- Midline location of primary tumor
- Stasis of lymph flow from a node completely replaced by tumor.

Sentinel lymph node identification and biopsy should be confirmed by a prospective randomized controlled trial before it may be considered a part of the standard of surgical care for vulvar carcinoma.

Management of a patient with positive groin nodes: After several observations, recommendations for the management of patients with positive groin nodes are as discussed further.

- Patients with one micrometastasis (metastatic deposit ≤5 mm diameter) should be observed after radical lymphadenectomy. The prognosis for this group of patients is excellent. Even if a unilateral groin dissection has been performed for a lateral lesion, there seems to be no indication for dissection of the other groin. Because contralateral lymph node involvement is likely only if there are multiple ipsilateral inguinal node metastases.[14,15] Dutch workers have reported no benefit for adjuvant radiation for patients with one positive node without extracapsular spread.[16]
- Patients with three or more micrometastases, one macrometastasis (>5 mm diameter), or any evidence of extracapsular spread should receive bilateral groin and pelvic radiation.
- There are insufficient data on patients with two micrometastases to draw definitive conclusions. If these patients are observed, it may be prudent to observe the contralateral groin with ultrasound for the first 6–12 months, if it has not been dissected.

Patients who undergo bilateral inguinofemoral lymphadenectomy as initial therapy and are found to have positive nodes, particularly more than one positive node are likely to benefit from postoperative irradiation to the groins and lower pelvis. Radiation therapy is superior to surgery in the management of patients with positive pelvic nodes. Several management options are available for patients found to have positive nodes; however, if postoperative radiotherapy to the inguinal nodes is deemed necessary, it would be reasonable to limit resection to grossly positive nodes. Excellent local control and minimal morbidity have been achieved when selective inguinal lymphadenectomy and tailored postoperative adjuvant therapy were administered to carefully selected patients.

ADVANCED STAGE DISEASE

Vulvar cancer may be considered advanced (stage III and IV) on the basis of the tumor's extension into the lower third of the urethra and vagina or the presence of bulky positive groin (inguinofemoral) nodes.

By definition, stage III tumor extends to the adjacent mucosal structures (urethral or vaginal orifices) or the inguinal lymph nodes.

Many of these tumors are bulky, although some are of small volume and considered as higher stage because of their proximity to critical structures such as the urethra, clitoris, vagina and anus. Some of these primary tumors can be curatively resected by radical operation like radical vulvectomy.

The tumor spreading to the anus, rectum, rectovaginal septum or bladder and proximal urethra some form of pelvic exenteration with radical vulvectomy can be done in these cases.

This type of operation can lead to perioperative mortality or postoperative complications like disfiguration, permanent colostomy, urinary diversion, psychological upset and many others.

Considering these grave complications, recent therapeutic efforts have focused on combined treatment modality which consists of sequenced radiation therapy or chemoradiation therapy and radical surgery. Preoperative chemoradiation therapy improves the surgical resection because modern chemoradiation therapy treatment has less side effects, and normal tissue damage and disfiguration is very less.

There are now ample data from retrospective and a few prospective trials from which it has been concluded that vulvar cancers, are radiosensitive and that function sparing operations are feasible in selected patients with advanced disease who receive combined modality treatment.

Commonly used preoperative chemotherapeutic agents are 5-fluorouracil (5-FU) and cisplatin. These agents act as radiosensitizers which enhance radiation effects.

Management of Advanced Stage Disease

For the management of advanced stage vulvar cancer patients should be individualized and a multidisciplinary team approach is desirable. As with early stage disease it is advantageous to determine the most appropriate treatment for:
- Primary tumor
- Groin and pelvic nodes.

Management of the Primary Tumor

If the tumor involves the distal vagina and/or urethral orifice and can be resected with clear surgical margins without need for a stoma, then primary surgical resection is the best option. Radical vulvectomy often will be required, although a modified radical vulvectomy to allow adequate clearance around the lesion while preserving some normal vulva may be appropriate.

Traditionally, the en bloc approach through a trapezoid or butterfly incision has been used[17] and this may be useful if there is extensive anterior disease. More commonly the separate incision approach is used, which involves using three separate incisions, one for the radical vulvectomy and one for each of the groin dissections.[18]

Technique for en block radical vulvectomy and groin dissection: The operation is usually performed with the patient in low lithotomy position. Vulvar groin dissection can proceed simultaneously with two teams of surgeons, if appropriate. The groin dissection has been described earlier.

The technique for radical vulvectomy: The traditional procedures for radical vulvectomy and bilateral lymphadenectomy described as a "butterfly" or "longhorn" approach have largely been abandoned. If the radical vulvectomy is performed through a separate incision, the lateral incision is elliptical. Each lateral incision should commence on the mons pubis anteriorly and extend through the fat and superficial fascia to the fascia over the pubic symphysis. It is easy to develop bluntly the plane immediately above the pubic symphysis and fascia lata. The skin incision is extended posteriorly along the labiocrural folds to the perianal area and extended down to the fascia lata.

The medial incision is placed to clear the tumor with margins of at least 1 cm. If necessary, the distal half of the urethra may be resected without compromising continence. If the tumor involves the urethra or vagina, dissection around the tumor is facilitated by transection of the vulva, thereby improving exposure of the involved area.

The specimen includes the bulbocavernosus muscles and the vestibular bulb. Because of the vascularity, it is desirable to perform most of the dissection by diathermy after the initial skin incision. The vessels supplying the clitoris should be clamped and tied, as should the posterolateral internal pudendal vessels.

Closure of large defects: It is usually possible to close the vulvar defect without tension. If a more extensive dissection has been required because of large primary lesion, a number of options are available to repair the defects.

- An area may be left open to granulate, which it usually does over a period of 6–8 weeks. This is particularly useful around the urethra, where sutures can cause urethral deviation and misdirection of the urinary stream.
- Full-thickness flaps may be devised.[19] An example is the rhomboid flap, which is best suited for covering large defects of the posterior vulva.
- Unilateral or bilateral gracilis myocutaneous grafts may be developed, these are the most useful when an extensive area from the mons pubis to the perianal area has been resected. Because the graft brings a new blood supply to the area, it is particularly applicable if the vulva is poorly vascularized from prior surgical resection or radiation.[20]
- If extensive defects exist in the groin and vulva, the tensor fascia lata myocutaneous graft may be applicable.

Management of the Groin and Pelvic Lymph Nodes

All patients with advanced vulvar cancer should have a detailed clinical examination and tomographic imaging of the groin, pelvis, and abdomen before surgery. Patients can be triaged into three groups, as follows:

1. *Patients with no clinically or radiologically suspicious nodes:* There are two possible approaches to these patients. They may be treated with bilateral inguinofemoral lymphadenectomy, performed through separate groin incisions. If there are two negative nodes, or up to two micrometastases (<5 mm tumor deposits) without extracapsular spread, the groins may be spared from any subsequent radiation fields. As with early stage disease, if there is one macrometastasis (>5 mm tumor deposit), three or more micrometastasis, or extracapsular spread, pelvic and groin radiation is indicated. An alternative approach that may be preferred in selected patients is to treat the groins with primary radiation, along with the vulvar lesion.
2. *Patients with clinically or radiologically suspicious resectable nodes:*
   – All enlarged groin nodes should be removed through a separate incision approach and sent for frozen-section diagnosis.

If metastatic disease is confirmed, a full lymphadenectomy should not be carried out.
- If the frozen section reveals no metastatic disease in the removed node, full groin dissection should be performed. Both disease-specific survival and groin recurrence-free intervals were superior in the group having nodal debulking, although with the small numbers in both series, the differences were not statistically significant.
- Full pelvic and groin irradiation should be given as soon as the groin incisions are healed, usually within 3 weeks.
- Any enlarged pelvic nodes seen in CT scan should be removed by extraperitoneal approach.
3. *Patients with fixed, unresectable groin nodes*: These patients should be treated with primary groin and pelvic radiation, probably in combination with chemotherapy. It may be appropriate to resect a residual groin mass following radiation if there is an incomplete response to radiation and no other evidence of metastatic disease.[21]

Management of patients for whom primary tumor involves the anus or proximal urethra:
Pelvic exenteration: When the primary disease involves the anus, rectum, rectovaginal septum, or proximal urethra, adequate surgical clearance of the primary tumor is possible only by some type of infralevator exenteration, (anterior, posterior or total), combined with radical vulvectomy and bilateral groin dissection. Such radical surgery is usually inappropriate for these patients; even if medically fit. For suitable surgical candidates, the psychological and postoperative morbidity are high. Nevertheless, a 5-year survival rate of approximately 50% can be expected with this approach. Spread to regional lymph nodes and complete resection are the most important prognostic factors following pelvic exenteration.[22]

Postoperative Management

In spite of the patients' age and compromised general medical health, the surgery for vulvar cancer is usually remarkably safe and complications are well tolerated. However postoperative mortality rate of about 1% can be expected, usually as a result of pulmonary embolism or myocardial infarction.

Management of postoperative period: Immediate postoperative management consists of frequent follow-up of general conditions for early diagnosis of a pulmonary embolism or myocardial infarction, or hemorrhage from operation site. Management in the subsequent days consists of:
- A low residue diet may be recommended on the first postoperative day.
- Bed rest is advisable for 2–3 days to allow immobilization of the wounds to help healing.
- A pneumatic calf compressor should be used to help prevent deep venous thrombosis.
- Prophylactic subcutaneous heparin or clexane should be used in the dose of 20–40 mg daily for 7–10 days for this purpose.
- Active, nonweight bearing leg movement should be encouraged to help prevent deep venous thrombosis.
- Perineal swab with povisep solution at least twice daily should be given until the patient is fully mobilized.
- When the patient is fully mobilized sitz baths or whirlpool therapy is helpful.
- A Foley catheter is usually left in the bladder until the patient is ambulant.
- Mild laxative can be given to prevent constipation.

Postoperative complications: The major perioperative immediate mortality related to the groin node dissection results from injury to the femoral vessels. Other causes of mortality are pulmonary embolism and myocardial infarction. The "triple incision" approach and sparing of all subcutaneous fat above the superficial fascia, has kept the incidence of woundbreak down very low. Patients who are heavy smoker and diabetic are at greatest risk. The most common problem is lymphocyst formation, which occurs in 40% of cases.[23] This seems to have become more common since the introduction of the practice of leaving the fascia lata over the muscles in the floor of the femoral triangle.

Management of large lymphocysts: Large lymphocysts are best managed by making a linear incision 1–2 cm long and inserting a corrugated drain until the skin flaps have adhered to the underlying tissues.

Prevention: Avoidance of early mobilization and long walks before the groin is completely healed.

Other early postoperative complications are:
- Cellulites
- Urinary tract infection
- Deep venous thrombosis
- Pulmonary embolism
- Myocardial infarction
- Hemorrhages
- Osteitis pubis (rare).

Late complications: The major late complication is chronic leg edema, which has been reported in as many as 69% of patients. According to a report of Royal Hospital for Women in Sydney, in about 50% of patients, the onset of lymphedema occurred within 3 months, while 85% experienced its onset within 12 months. Lymphedema was significantly related to the occurrence of early complication, particularly cellulitis.[24]

The second most common late complication is recurrent lymphangitis or cellulitis of the leg which occurs in 10% of the patients. It may develop very quickly as an acute emergency and the patient may need hospitalization and intravenous antibiotics.

Other late complications are: Urinary stress incontinence, with or without genital prolapse, occurs in about 10% of patients and may require corrective surgery.
- Chronic urinary tract infection results from prolonged catheterization and may require repeated use of antibiotics.
- Introital stenosis can lead to dyspareunia and may require a vertical relaxing incision repaired by a transverse suture.
- An uncommon late complication is femoral hernia which can easily be prevented during surgery by closure of the femoral canal with a suture from the inguinal ligament to the cooper ligament.
- Pubic osteomyelitis and rectovaginal or rectoperineal fistula are rare late complications.

ROLE OF RADIATION THERAPY IN VULVAR CANCER

Radiation therapy is playing an increasingly important role in the management of patients with vulvar cancer, but a "Patterns of Care" study among members of the Gynecologic Cancer Intergroup revealed differences in the indications for treatment, treatment fields, and use of chemotherapy between groups.[25] This was thought to be due to the rarity of the disease, and the lack of randomized trials.

Following initial resection of a primary vulvar tumor, various surgicopathologic features have been identified that are associated with a higher risk of local recurrences. These features are:
- Tumor size
- Nodal status
- Margin status
- Lymphovascular space invasion
- Deep tumor invasion.

Many local recurrences are controlled with additional surgery or irradiation, surgery for local recurrences is often morbid. Moreover local recurrences may provide additional opportunity for regional or distant metastasis. Adjuvant radiation of the primary tumor bed after surgery in selected patients with close margin or other high-risk features may improve the local tumor control.

The indications for radiation therapy in patients with vulvar cancer are still evolving. At present radiation seems to be clearly indicated in the following situations:
- For patients with advanced disease who are indicated for pelvic exenteration. Data indicate that high complete response rates can be achieved with radiation therapy, with or without chemotherapy. High local control rates have been achieved in selected patients with 40–50 Gy followed by organ sparing surgery. In cases where surgery is still risky for organ dysfunction, radiation alone may be the initial treatment of choice, reserving radical surgery for local recurrences. With the experience gained from preoperative radiation with or without concurrent chemotherapy, it should be regarded as the treatment of choice for patients with advanced vulvar cancer who would otherwise require some type of pelvic exenteration.

- After surgery, to treat the pelvic lymph nodes and groins in patients with more than two micrometastases, one macrometastasis, or extracapsular spread.
- After surgery, to help prevent local recurrence and improve survival in patients with involved surgical margins (>5 mm). For patients who had close surgical margins, radiation gives significantly better local control but no survival benefit.

Possible roles for radiation therapy include the following:
- As primary therapy for patients with small primary tumors, particularly clitoral or periclitoral lesions in young and middle-aged women, in whom surgical resection would have significant psychological consequences.
- As an alternative to groin dissection in patients with no lymph nodes. Several retrospective clinical reviews have suggested that radiation alone can control microscopic nodal disease if adequate coverage of the inguinal and femoral nodes is confirmed.

Concurrent Chemoradiation Therapy

In 1989, Thomas et al.[26] was the first to report on the use of chemoradiation for patients with advanced vulvar cancer. Several subsequent studies have reported that complete pathologic response rates of between 31% and 55% can be achieved in these patients, even with modest doses of radiation. However, the pathologic response rates seen with chemoradiation were not obviously superior to those achieved with radiation alone.

Alternatively, in patients who present with more advanced primary tumors, radiation therapy may be delivered preoperatively. Several investigators have reported excellent responses and high local control rates after preoperative treatment of advanced tumor with relatively modest doses of radiation therapy followed by local resection. A number of published series have suggested the therapeutic benefit of concurrent chemoradiation, typically followed by limited surgical resection, in addressing locally advanced disease. Randomized trials of the role of chemoradiation, have not been done in vulvar cancer. Recent trials demonstrated improved local control and survival when concurrent cisplatin-containing chemotherapy was added to radiation treatment of cervical cancer, suggesting that this approach may be useful for women with other locally advanced lower genital tract neoplasms.

Radiation Therapy Technique

Techniques commonly used for the treatment of vulvar carcinoma reflect the need to encompass the lower pelvic and inguinal nodes as well as the vulva while minimizing the dose to femoral heads. One approach is to employ an anterior field that encompasses the inguinal regions, lower pelvic nodes, and vulva and a narrower posterior field that encompasses the lower pelvic nodes and vulva but excludes the majority of the femoral heads. CT scans are used to determine the appropriate electron energy and to detect enlarged nodes that may not be appreciated on clinical exam. Gross disease in the groins or vulva may be boosted with en face electron fields. In some cases, interstitial implants or face electron fields may be used to boost the dose at the primary site. If radiation is directed only to the regional nodes, with intentional sparing of vulva, care must be taken to avoid a large "midline" block, which may lead to higher medial groin and vulvar failures.

The complex anatomy of the vulva and its regional lymphatics, interwoven with critical adjacent normal tissues, has led some investigators to propose the use of intensity modulated radiation (IMR) therapy in the management of vulvar cancer.

Acute Complications of Radiation Therapy

Acute radiation reactions are brisk, and doses of 35–45 Gy routinely induce confluent moist desquamation of skin. With adequate local care, this acute reaction usually heals within 3–4 weeks. Sitz baths, steroid cream, and treatment of possible superimposed *Candida* infection all help to minimize the discomfort. If the patient is sufficiently flexible, she may be placed in a frog leg position during treatment to minimize the dose and ensuing skin reaction on the medial thighs; care must be taken to deliver an adequate dose to vulvar skin. Although most patients will develop confluent mucositis by the fourth week of treatment. This is usually tolerated if the patient is warned in advance and assured that the discomfort will resolve after treatment is completed. Although a treatment break is occasionally required, delays should be minimized, because they may allow time for repopulation of tumor cells.

Late Complication of Radiation Therapy

Many factors add to the late morbidity of radiation treatment in patients with vulvar carcinoma. Patients with advanced vulvar carcinomas often are treated with radiation therapy following radical surgery, which may include extensive dissection of the inguinal and possible pelvic nodes. Large ulcerative cutaneous lesions frequently have superimposed infections, such as diabetes multiple prior surgeries, and osteoporosis. The contribution of concurrent chemotherapy to local morbidity is not yet clearly defined, but may contribute to bowel and bone complications.

The incidence of lower extremity edema after inguinal irradiation alone is negligible. Although radiation therapy probably contributes to the incidence of peripheral edema following radical nodes dissection, no difference was evident in a Gynecologic Oncology Group (GOG) randomized study. With careful treatment planning technique, the risk of major late complication following regional nodal radiation, either electively or adjuvant to lymph node dissection is low.

Chemotherapy in Vulvar Cancer

Squamous cell carcinoma is the only histological type of vulvar cancer for which reproducible information exists on the value of cytotoxic therapy. Several drugs have been tested by phase II clinical trial in squamous cell vulvar cancer. From phase II clinical trials it has become obvious that only doxorubicin and bleomycin appear to have activity as single agents. Cisplatin has very little activity in vulvar and vaginal squamous cell carcinoma.

Neoadjuvant Chemotherapy in Vulvar Cancer

In 2006, a study from Indianapolis reported the use of neoadjuvant chemotherapy for patients whose vulvar cancer involved the anus and or utethra.[27] Ten patients received cisplatin and 5-FU, and three received cisplatin alone. Patients receiving cisplatin alone showed no measurable response, while all patients receiving cisplatin and

5-FU achieved at least a partial response. With median follow-up of 49 months (3-90 months) nine patients receiving cisplatin and 5-FU followed by surgery remained disease free.

A prospective, multicenter study of neoadjuvant chemotherapy for locally advanced vulvar cancer was reported from Buenos Aires in 2012.[28] Thirty-five patients were recruited to the study, and a variety of different chemotherapeutic regimens were used. Twenty-seven patients (77%) underwent radical surgery, including two who required posterior exenteration for persistent rectal involvement. Twenty-four patients (68%) were without evidence of disease, with a median follow-up of 49 months (range 4-155 months).

Concurrent Cisplatin-based Chemotherapy

With the results obtained with concurrent cisplatin-based chemotherapy and radiation therapy in locally advanced squamous cancer of cervix, one must consider a similar approach in the patient with locally advanced squamous cell cancer of vulva. Several drug combinations have been used in squamous vulvar cancer. Toxicity with these drug regimens has been reported as tolerable.

In advanced inoperable diseases, concomitant use of cytotoxic therapy with irradiation has been reported. The largest experience in vulvar cancer has been reported be GOG.

RECURRENT VULVAR CANCER

Most treatment failures are diagnosed within 2 years, and in patients with early disease, most recurrences are on the vulva. Distant metastases do occur, particularly in the presence of multiple lymph node metastases.

Local recurrence at a site distant from the primary tumor (which could be considered a new primary lesion), had a good prognosis, 66.7% of patients surviving 3 years. By contrast survival after recurrence at the primary tumor site was poor, only 15.4% of patients surviving 3 years. None of seven patients with skin bridge recurrence was alive at 1 year.

Local vulvar recurrences are usually amenable to further surgical resection. A variety of plastic surgical techniques may facilitate adequate surgical resection, particularly for large recurrences. Myocutaneous graft which may be used include the gluteal thigh flap, the rectus abdominous flap, the gracilis flap, and the tensor fascia lata flap.

Radiation therapy has been used to treat vulvar recurrences. When brachytherapy is used in this region, great care must be taken not to have radiation sources close to vulvar skin or mucous membranes, because the dose of radiation close to interstitial needles can be 5–10 times greater than the prescribed dose. For this reason, and because patients treated with brachytherapy for vulvar cancer are reported to have high rates of necrosis, many gynecologic radiation oncologists avoid its use in this region. Modern conformal external beam radiation techniques, such as intensity-modulated radiotherapy (IMRT) deliver a more homogenous dose to vulvovaginal target tissues, and would be expected to have a much lower risk of necrosis; however, few data specific to locally recurrent disease treated are available.

Regional and distant recurrences are difficult to manage.[29] Although survival rates are low, some patients are cured with surgery and regional radiation therapy. Chemotherapeutic agents that have activity against squamous carcinomas may be offered for distant metastases. The most active agents are cisplatin, methotrexate, cyclophosphamide, bleomycin, and mitomycin C, but response rates are low and the duration of response is usually disappointing.

Recently a targeted therapy was used for the first time in patients with vulvar cancer. The epidermal growth factor receptor (EGFR) inhibitor, erlotinib, was used in 41 patients, 11 (27.5%) of whom had a partial response and 16 (40%) had stable disease. Responses were of short duration, but toxicities were acceptable.

Prognosis

With appropriate management, the prognosis for vulvar cancer is generally good, the overall 5-year survival rate in operable cases being approximately 70%. Survival correlates with the 1988 FIGO clinical stage of disease (Table 5.3) and with lymph node status.

In the 26th FIGO annual report, patients with negative lymph nodes had a 5-year survival rate of 80.7%; the survival rate fell to 13.3% for patients with four or more positive nodes.[33]

TABLE 5.3: 5-year survival versus International Federation of Gynecology and Obstetrics (FIGO) clinical stage for patients with curative intent.[30-32]

FIGO clinical stage	Corrected 5-year survival
I	90.4
II	77.1
III	51.3
IV	18
Total	69.7

The number of positive groin nodes is the single most important prognostic variable and the survival rates for patients with positive pelvic nodes are only about 11%. Patients with one microscopically positive node have a good prognosis, but patients with three or more positive nodes have a poor prognosis. Extracapsular spread is a poor prognostic factor.

More than three inguinal node involvements have a high incidence of positive pelvic nodes. There is evidence that many patients with pelvic node metastases can be cured if they receive postoperative or definitive radiation therapy. Microscopic pelvic node metastases are rarely detected today because elective pelvic node dissections are rarely performed.

A review of patients treated with definitive radiation therapy for grossly involved pelvic lymph nodes demonstrated an overall 5-year survival rate of 43%, despite extensive locoregional disease. These data suggest that patients with regional disease confined to the groin and distal pelvis should be treated with curative intend whenever possible.

There is often a tendency to undertreat patients over the age of 80, on the false assumption that these patients will die of other diseases before their cancer recurs. It is a fundamental error to treat patients on the basis of chronologic rather than biologic age, and British workers reported a 25% recurrence rate for patients with vulvar cancer over 80 years of age treated according to their standard protocol, compared to a 53.5% recurrence rate when there was a protocol violation.[34]

Overall prognosis of squamous cell type vulvar cancer depends on the following factors:
- *Size of the tumor:* The larger the size of the tumor, the poorer the prognosis.

- *Location of the tumor:* The deeper and more medial the location of the tumor, the lower the 5-year survival rate.
- *Stage of the disease:* The higher the stage, the poorer the prognosis.
- *Lymph node metastases:* The higher the number of lymph nodes involved, the poorer the prognosis. When no node is involved, 5-year survival rate is 90% but when only one node is involved, the 5-year survival rate is 40%.

Results of Therapy

The overall results of therapy for women with squamous cell cancers of the vulva are excellent. Approximately two-thirds of patients present with early-stage tumors and 5-year survival rates of 80–90% are routine. For patients with advanced disease 5-year survival rates are poor: 60% for stage III cases and 15% for stage IV. The survival rate for women with nodal spread is one-half that of women without nodal disease who have similarly sized primary tumors.

Follow-up

Patients with vulvar cancer should be seen every 3 months for 2 years, every 6 months for 5 years, and at least annually for life. Data from the Mayo Clinic have shown that in 35% of cases, vulvar cancer recurs 5 years or more after diagnosis. Virtually all these late recurrences are on the vulva, and many start as in situ disease, which can often be resected in the office under local anesthesia if diagnosed early. Patients should be taught self-examination, and told to seek attention if they develop vulvar irritation or visual change.

VERRUCOUS CARCINOMA

Verrucous carcinomas are a variant of squamous cell carcinoma that occurs in postmenopausal women. They are most commonly found in the oral cavity, but may be found on any moist membrane composed of squamous epithelium. They are a distinct entity, with no association with HPV infection, and a peculiar distribution pattern of cytokeratins AEI and AE3 on immunohistochemical stain.

These tumors are large fungating cauliflower-like masses, the diameter of which ranges from 1–15 cm. Microscopically these tumors contain multiple papillary fronds that lack the central connective tissue case, which are the characteristics of condylomata acuminate. The gross and microscopic features of verrucous carcinoma are very similar to these of the giant condyloma of Buschke Lowenstein, and they probably represent the same disease entity. Adequate biopsy of the base of the lesion is required to differentiate a verrucous carcinoma from benign condylomata accuminata or a squamous cell carcinoma with verrucous growth pattern.

Clinically these are slowly growing but locally destructive lesions. Even bone marrow may be invaded. VIN or invasive squamous cell carcinoma may be seen in association with verrucous carcinoma. Although lymph node metastasis is exceedingly rare, local destruction and tumor recurrence are common.

Treatment of Verrucous Carcinoma

Radical local excision is the standard treatment. Enlarged lymph nodes are usually caused by inflammation, but metastasis should be excluded by fine needle aspiration cytology or excision biopsy.

Radiation therapy is contraindicated because it may induce anaplastic transformation with subsequent regional and distant metastasis. Recurrent cases need surgical excision in the form of some type of exenteration.

REFERENCES

1. Hellman K, Silfversward C, Nilsson B, et al. Primary carcinoma of the vagina: Factors influencing the age at diagnosis. The Radium hemmet series 1956-1996. Int J Gynecol Cancer. 2004;14(3):491-501.
2. Berek JS, Hacker NF. Berek & Hacker's Gynecologic Oncology, 6th edition. Philadelphia: Wolters Kluwer; 2014.
3. Benedet JL, Murphy KJ, Fairey RN, et al. Primary invasive carcinoma of the vagina. Obstet Gynecol. 1983;62:715-9.
4. Ball HG, Berman ML. Management of primary vaginal carcinoma. Gynecol Oncol. 1982;14:154-63.
5. Peters W, Kumar N, Morley G. Carcinoma of the vagina. Factors influencing outcome. Cancer. 1985;55;892-7.
6. Sulak P, Barnhill D, Heller P, et al. Nonsquamous cancer of the vagina. Gynecol Oncol. 1988;29:309-20.

7. Dalbagni G, Donat SM, Eschwege P, et al. Results of high dose rate brachytherapy, anterior pelvic exenteration and external beam radiotherapy for carcinoma of the female urethra. J Urol. 2001;166:1759-61.
8. Helmman K, Lundell M, Silfversward C, et al. Clinical and histopathologic factors related to prognosis in primary squamous cell carcinoma of the vagina. Int. J Gynecol Cancer. 2006;16:1201-11.
9. Thyavhally YB, Wuntkal R, Bakshi G, et al. Primary carcinoma of the female urethra: Single center experience of 18 cases. JPN J Clin Oncol. 2005;35:84-7.
10. Jones RW, Matthews JH. Early clitoral carcinoma successfully treated by radiotherapy and bilateral inguinal lymphadenectomy. Int J Hynecol Cancer. 1999;9:348-50.
11. Nicklin JL, Hacker NF, Heintze SW, et al. An anatomical study of inguinal lymph node topography and clinical implications for the surgical management of vulval cancer. Int Gynecol Cancer. 1995;5:128-33.
12. Micheletti L, Levi AC, Bogliatto F et al. Radionale and definition of the lateral extension of the inguinal lymphadenectomy for vulvar cancer drived from an embryological and anatomical study. J Surg Oncol. 2002;81:19-24.
13. Micheletti L, Borgno G, Barbero M, et al. Deep femoral lymphadenectomy with preservation of the fascia lata. Preliminary report on 42 invasive vulvar varcinomas. J Reprod Med. 1990;35:1130-3.
14. Homesley HD, BN, Sedlis A, et al. Radiation therapy versus pelvic node resection for carcinoma of the vulva with positive groin nodes. Obstet Gynecol. 1986;68:733-40.
15. Gonzalez Bosquet J, Magrina JF, Magrina, JF et al. Patterns of inguinal groin metastases in squamous cell carcinoma of the vulva. Gynecol Oncol. 2007;105:742-6.
16. Fons G, Groenen SM, Oonk MH, et al. Adjuvant radiotherapy in patients with vulvar cancer and intra capsular lymph node metastasis is not beneficial. Gynecol Oncol. 2009;114:343-5.
17. Morley GW. Infiltrative carcinoma of the vulva: results of surgical treatment. Am J Obstet Gynecol. 1976;124:874-88.
18. Hacker NF, Leuchter RS, Berek JS, et al. Radical vulvectomy and bilateral inguinal lymphadenectomy through separate groin incisions. Obstet Gynecol. 1981;58:574-9.
19. Low JJ, Hacker NF. Vulvar reconstruction in gynecologic oncology. Hung J Gynecol Oncol. 1999;3:105-12.
20. Ballon SC, Donaldon RC, Roberts JA, et al. Reconstruction of the vulva using a myocutaneous graft. Gynecol Oncol. 1979;7:123-7.

21. Montana GS, Thomas GM, Moore DH, et al. Preoperative chemoradiation for carcinoma of vulva with N2/N3 nodes: A gynecologic oncology group study. Int J Radiat Oncol Biol Phys. 2000;48:1007-13.
22. Forner DM, Lampe B. Exenteration in the treatment of Stage III/IV vulvar cancer. Gynecol Oncol. 20012;124:87-91.
23. Gaarenstrom KN, Kenter GG, Trimbos JB, et al. Postoperative complications after vulvectomy and inguinofemoral lymphadenectomy using separate groin incisions. Int J Gynecol Cancer. 2003;13:522-7.
24. Ryan M, Stainton MC, Slaytor EK, et al. Aetiology and prevalence of lower limb lymphoedema following treatment for gynecological cancer. Aust N Z J Obstet Gynecol. 2003;43:148-51.
25. Gaffney DK, Du Bois A, Narayan K, et al. Patterns of care for radiotherapy in vulvar cancer: a Gynecologic Cancer Intergroup study. Int J Gynecol Cancer. 2009;19:163-7.
26. Thomas G, Dembo A, Depetrillo A, et al. Concurrent radiation and chemotherapy in vulvar cancer carcinoma. Gynecol. 1989;34:263-7.
27. Geisler JP, Manahan KJ, Buller RF. Neoadjuvant chemotherapy in vulvar cancer: Avoiding primary exenteration. Gynecol Oncol. 2006;100:53-7.
28. Aragona AM, Cuneo N, Soderini AH, et al. Tailoring the treatment of locally advanced squamous cell carcinoma of the vulva: neoadjuvant chemotherapy followed by radical surgery: results from a multicenter study. Int J Gynecol Cancer. 2012;22:1258-63.
29. Podratz KC, Symmonds RE, Taylor WF. Carcinoma of the vulva: Analysis of treatment failures. Am J Obstet Gynecol. 1982;143:340-51.
30. Benedet JL, Turko M, Fairey RN, et al. Squamous carcinoma of the vulva: results of treatment, 1938 to 1976. Am J Obstet Gynecol. 1979;134:201-7.
31. Hacker NF, Berek JS, Lagasse LD, et al. Management of regional lymph nodes and their prognostic influence in vulvar cancer. Obstet Gynecol. 1983:61:408-12.
32. Cavangh D, Roberts WS, Bryson SC, et al. Changing trends in the surgical treatment of invasive carcinoma of the vulva. Surg Gynecol Obstet. 1986;162:164-8.
33. Thaker N, Klopp AH, Jhingran A, et al. Survival outcomes for patients with pelvic lymph node-positive Stage IVB vulvar cancer: Time to reconsider the FIGO staging system? Int J Radiat Oncol Biol Phys. 2013;87:S129.
34. Talat A, Brinkmann D, Nagar Y et al. Experience in the management of patients older than 80 years with vulvar cancer. Int Gynecol Cancer. 2009;19:752-5.

CHAPTER 6

Nonsquamous Type of Vulvar Cancer

VULVAR MALIGNANT MELANOMA

Nine (9%) of all primary malignant neoplasms of vulva and 3% of all melanomas in women are malignant melanoma. These tumors occur predominantly in Caucasian women, and the mean age at diagnosis is 55 years of age. Although 75% are pigmented, 25% are nonpigmented amelanotic melanomas, which resemble vulvar squamous cell carcinoma.

Sites of Origin
- Labia minora
- Clitoris.

Spread
- Superficial spread to the urethra and vagina
- Primary spread to lymphatics
- Satellite lesions are found.

Naked Eye Appearance of Malignant Melanoma of Vulva

Non-pigmented lesions closely resemble invasive squamous cell carcinoma of vulva. Pigmented lesions have special characteristics similar to nevi. All nevi of the vulva are of the junctional variety.

These are raised lesions at the mucocutaneous junction (Figs. 6.1 and 6.2).

There are three basic histologic types: (1) the *superficial spreading melanoma*, which tends to remain relatively superficial early in its development; (2) the *mucosal lentiginous melanoma*, a flat freckle, which may become quite extensive but tends to remain superficial; and (3) the *nodular melanoma*, which is a raised lesion that penetrates deeply and may metastasize widely. A Swedish study of 219 cases reported that the mucosal lentiginous melanoma was the most frequent type (57%).[1]

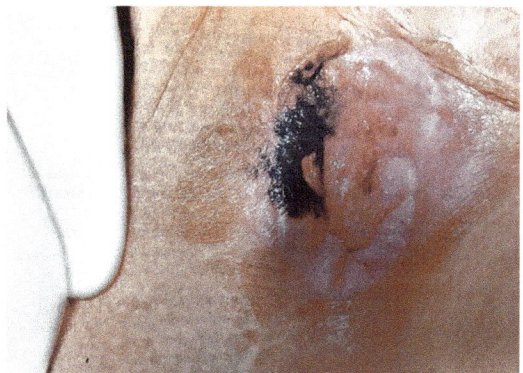

Fig. 6.1: Malignant melanoma—dark black color.

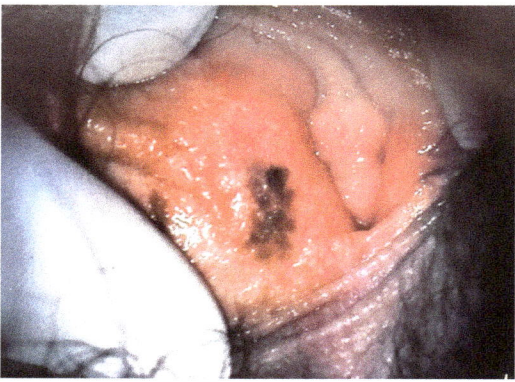

Fig. 6.2: Benign melanoma—variable color.

Diagnosis

All pigmented lesions of the vulva should be suspected for malignant melanoma of the vulva and an excision biopsy should be taken with a 0.5-1 cm of normal skin margin.

The level of invasion and tumor thickness are essential measurements in evaluating malignant melanoma. Risk of metastasis depends on tumor thickness and other factors. The prognosis for malignant melanoma of the vulva is classified in the following way:

Tumor Thickness

- Less than 0.75 mm—no risk of metastasis
- Up to 1 mm thickness—minimal risk
- Less than 1.94 mm thickness—good prognosis
- More than 2 mm thickness or mitotic count $10/mm^2$—poor prognosis
- Minimum or nil inflammatory reaction—poor prognosis
- Surface ulceration—poor prognosis.

Vulvar melanomas are a rare type of vulvar malignancy, most commonly arising de novo, but from a preexisting junctional nevus. Predominantly they are found in postmenopausal Caucasian women, and commonly on the labia minora or the clitoris.

According to the SEER database from 1973-2008, compared to cutaneous melanomas, patients with vulvar vaginal melanomas were more likely to be older (68 vs 52 years; $p<0.0001$) and to present with advanced disease (8.4% vs 2.7%; $p<0.008$).

Staging

The International Federation of Gynecology and Obstetrics (FIGO) staging used for squamous cell lesions is not applicable for melanomas because these lesions are usually much smaller and the prognosis is related to the depth of penetration rather than to the diameter of the lesion.

A revised American Joint Committee on Cancer (AJCC) Staging System for cutaneous melanomas came in to effect in 2002 (Table 6.1).

Prognostic factors taken into account include:
- Primary tumor thickness (replacing level of invasion)
- Ulceration

TABLE 6.1: Revised 2002 American Joint Committee on Cancer (AJCC) staging for cutaneous melanoma.

Stage	Primary tumor	Lymph node(N)	Metastases (M)
0	In situ (Tis)	No nodes	None
IA	<1 mm no ulceration/ Clark's II and III (T1a)	No nodes	None
IB	<1 mm+ ulceration Clark's IV and V ((T1b) 1.01–2 mm no ulceration	No nodes	None
IIA	1.01–2 mm + ulceration (T2b) 2.01–4 mm no ulceration (T3a)	No nodes	None
IIB	2.01–4 mm + ulceration (T3b) >4 mm no ulceration	No nodes	None
IIC	> 4 mm + ulceration (T4b)	No nodes	None
IIIA	Any thickness, no ulceration	1 node micro metastasis (n1 a)	
IIIB	Any thickness, with ulceration Any thickness , no ulceration Any thickness, ± ulceration	1 node micro metastasis (n1 a) Up to 3 nodes micrometastases (n2a) In-transit met/satellite + positive nodes (n2c)	None
IIIC	Any thickness, with ulceration Any thickness, ± ulceration	Up to 3 nodes macrometastases (n2b) ≥ metastatic nodes/matted nodes/ in-transit With positive nodes (n3)	None
IV	Any thickness	Any nodes	Present

- Number of metastatic lymph nodes
- Micrometastatic disease based on sentinel lymph node biopsy or elective node dissection
- Site/sites of distant disease
- Serum lactate dehydrogenase level.

Management of Vulvar Malignant Melanoma
- Management of the primary lesions
- Management of the groin lymph nodes.

Management of the Primary Lesions

It has become apparent from several small series that the same surgical principles that apply to cutaneous melanomas should be applied for the treatment of vulvar melanomas.[2]

More conservative surgery has been commenced for cutaneous melanomas. In the 1980s and although vulvar melanomas carry a much worse of prognosis this trend has been followed.[3,4]

A multicenter study in the United States of 77 patients in 2011[2] and a Mayo clinic report of 36 patients on 2013[5] confirmed the validity of conservative vulvar resection as for squamous lesion.

As melanomas typically involve the clitoris and labia minora, the vulvo-urethral margin of the resection is the most common site of failure.

It is necessary that the distal urethra may have to be resected in order to obtain an inner margin of at least 1 cm.

Podratz et al. demonstrated a 10-year survival rate of 61% for lateral lesions, compared to 37% for medial lesions (p <0.027).[6]

Management of the Groin Lymph Nodes

According to the authors of *Berek and Hacker's Gynecology Oncology*, current policy is to perform a radical local excision with 1 cm margins for the primary lesion. In patients with more than 1 mm of stromal invasion, at least an ipsilateral inguinofemoral lymphadenectomy is performed. Sentinel node biopsy is reserved for the few patients who do not want to take the 50–60% risk of developing lymphedema.

Adjuvant Therapy

Interferon alpha 2b (IFN-α-2b) was the first agent to show significant value as an adjuvant treatment for melanoma in a randomized controlled trial.[7]

Prognosis

Results of the treatment of vulvar melanomas are quite unpredictable but the overall prognosis is poor. The mean 5-year survival rate for reported cases of vulvar melanoma ranges from 21.7% (198) to 54%.[1] Patients with lesions invading to 1 mm or less have an excellent prognosis, but as the depth of invasion increases, the prognosis worsens (Chung et al.).[8]

BARTHOLIN'S GLAND CARCINOMA

Most common primary adenocarcinomas of the vulva arise within the Bartholin's gland. Only 1% of vulvar carcinoma arises from the Bartholin's gland. 50% of these carcinomas are of the squamous cell type and the other 50% are adenocarcinoma. Paget's disease can give rise to adenocarcinoma type adenosquamous carcinoma and transitional cell carcinoma. Carcinoma of the Bartholin's gland generally occurs in older women and is rare in women younger than 50 years of age.

Primary carcinoma of the Bartholin's gland accounts for approximately 5% of vulvar malignancies. It is a very rare tumor and individual experience is low. So guided management mostly depends on a review of the literature.

The bilateral Bartholin's glands are also called greater vestibular glands situated posterolaterally in the vulva, deep to the labia majora. Their main duct is lined by stratified squamous epithelium, which changes to transitional epithelium as the terminal ducts are reached. The gland itself is lined by columnar epithelium. Because the tumors may arise from the gland or the ducts, a variety of histological types may occur, including adenocarcinomas, squamous carcinomas which cover almost 98% of these carcinomas.

Paget's disease of the vulva can give rise to adenocarcinoma, adenosquamous carcinoma, transitional cell carcinoma and adenoid cystic carcinomas.

Carcinoma of the Bartholin's gland usually occurs in older women and is rare in women younger than 50 years of age. So, in women age 50 and older or when palpable lesions persist, after drainage excision of the Bartholin's glands rather than drainage is recommended.

To classify a vulvar tumor as a Bartholin's gland tumor some criteria must be fulfilled. These criteria are as follows:
- The tumor is in the correct anatomical position
- The tumor is located deep in the labium majus
- The overlying skin is intact
- Some recognizable glandular tissue is present.

Strict adherence to these criteria may result in under diagnosis. Bartholin's gland carcinomas are often misdiagnosed as Bartholin's gland cysts or abscesses. Other differential diagnoses of any para rectovaginal neoplasm should include cloacogenic carcinoma and secondary neoplasm.

The adenoid cystic variety if Bartholin's gland carcinoma accounts for approximately 10%. It is a slowly growing tumor with a marked propensity for perineural and local invasion. The perineural infiltration is quite characteristic and may account for the pruritus and burning sensation that is experienced by many patients before a palpable mass is evident.

Diagnosis

Diagnoses of Bartholin's gland carcinomas are very difficult because
- The gland is very deeply seated
- Very difficult to differentiate between benign and malignant tumor by examination
- Very difficult to excise the whole of the Bartholin's cyst
- Always need biopsy to diagnose malignancy as very difficult to detect in their early growth.

In clinical practice, it is generally advisable to excise an enlarged Bartholin's gland in a woman aged 50 or more, especially if there is no known history of prior Bartholin's cyst. If a palpable mass persists after the cyst is drained, an excision is indicated.

Spreading

The tumor spreads to the rectum or ischiorectal fossa by a direct route. Lymphatic spread may occur to the deep pelvic lymph nodes. Approximately 20% of women with primary carcinoma of the Bartholin's gland have metastatic tumor to the inguinofemoral lymph nodes at the time of primary diagnosis.

Treatment of Bartholin's Gland Carcinoma

If the tumor does not involve the surrounding structures, it should be treated by radical resection of the primary tumor and ipsilateral inguinofemoral lymphadenectomy. Sometimes an extensive dissection of the ischiorectal fossa is required and this may be facilitated by performing block resection of the primary lesion and the groin.

If the ipsilateral groin nodes are positive for malignancy, bilateral groin and pelvic node radiation may be indicated. According to a study at the MD Anderson Hospital, postoperative radiation decreases the likelihood of local recurrence from 27% to 7%.[9]

This mode of surgery is applicable to adenoid cystic carcinomas and adjuvant radiation is recommended for positive margins or perineural invasion.

According to the author from Massachusetts General Hospital chemoradiation is an effective alternative to surgery.

Indications for primary chemoradiation or neoadjuvent chemotherapy are:
- If the tumor is fixed to the inferior pubic ramus
- It involves adjacent structures, such as the anal sphincter or rectum, in order to avoid exenterative surgery.

Prognosis

Because of the deep location of the gland, cases tend to be more advanced than squamous cell carcinomas at the time of diagnosis, but stage for stage, the prognosis is similar.

Adenoid cystic tumors are less likely to metastasize to lymph nodes and carry a somewhat better prognosis. However, late recurrences may occur in the lungs, liver, or bone, so 10- and 15-year survival rates are more appropriate when evaluating these tumors.[10,11]

BASAL CELL CARCINOMA

It is the most common skin cancer, 85% of which occur in the head and neck region. As with melanomas, its incidence can be strongly related with sun exposure. According to study done at University of Florence, Italy, it is the second most common vulvar cancer after squamous cell carcinoma of the vulva.

About 1–2% of vulvar carcinomas may be of basal cell origin. Macroscopic appearance of the tumor may be of three types:
1. Papillomatous or elevated lesions
2. Pigmented moles
3. Simple pruritic maculopapular eruption.

The tumor originates from the primordial basal cells of the epidermis or hair follicles. So, it arises exclusively from labia majora.

Characteristics

As with other basal cell carcinomas, vulvar lesions appear as a "rodent ulcer" with rolled edges. It is a slow growing, locally infiltrating, and deeply penetrating indolent ulcer. Grossly these appear as flesh colored to whitish nodules or plaques that are often ulcerated.

The presentation is variable. The lesions may simulate inflammatory dermatosis, such as eczema or psoriasis, or as an infectious process such as chronic candidiasis. Any inflammatory lesion not responding to usual treatment should arouse suspicions of basal cell carcinoma. Most lesions are less than 2 cm in diameter, but giant lesions may occasionally occur.

They occur most commonly in post-menopausal Caucasian women and pruritus is the most common complaint. Treatment with local excision is usually adequate. Lymphatic or distant spread is exceedingly rare.

- These are moderately radiosensitive, so radiation may be useful in selected cases.
- Prognosis is good, despite roughly a 20% risk of local recurrence.

PAGET'S DISEASE AND OTHER VULVAR ADENOCARCINOMAS

Vulvar Paget's disease typically presents as an eczematoid red, weeping area on the vulva, often localized to the labia majora, perianal body, clitorial area and other sites. This disease typically occurs in older, postmenopausal Caucasian (white, light and older) women and may be associated with an underlying primary adenocarcinoma. Invasive Paget's disease of 1 mm or less in depth of invasion has reportedly little risk of recurrence.

Adenocarcinomas of the vulva usually arise in a Bartholin's gland or in association with Paget's disease. They may rarely arise from the skin appendages, paraurethral glands, minor vestibular glands, aberrant breast tissue, endometriosis or a misplaced cloacal remnant. A particularly aggressive type is the adenosquamous carcinoma.

Paget's disease of the vulva is rare. Most affected patients are in their seventh or eighth decade of life and experience local irritation, pruritus, and bleeding. The lesion has slightly raised edges and is erythematous, with islands of white epithelium (Fig. 6.3). Lesions are multifocal, sharply demarcated and often have foci of excoriation and induration. Adenocarcinoma of the underlying sweat glands is found in 10-15% of patients who have intraepithelial Paget's disease. In addition, 10% of patients with vulvar Paget's disease are found to have associated breast or genitourinary cancer; this workup should include colonoscopy, cystoscopy, mammogram, and colposcopy. If the disease is limited to the epithelium, its clinical course is usually prolonged and indolent

This is the microscopic appearance of Paget disease. The Paget cells are large and have abundant cytoplasm and a large nucleous. Most of the Paget cells are in the basal layer of the epithelium. However, two Paget cells are seen near the surface (upper right). Parakeratosis is seen above these cells (Fig. 6.4).

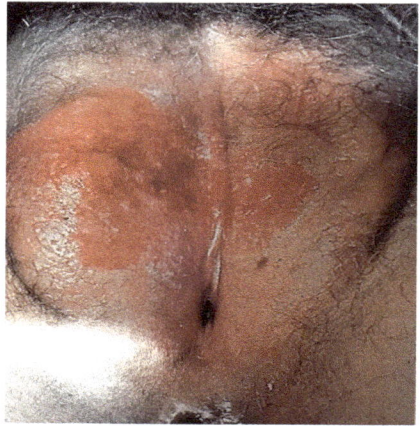

Fig. 6.3: Paget's disease of vulva.

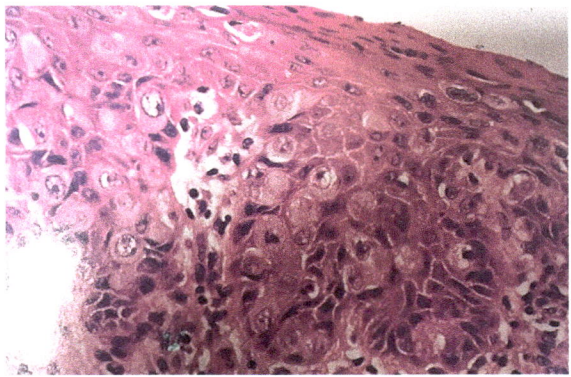

Fig. 6.4: Microscopic appearance of Paget's disease.

Treatment

Although radical surgery was formerly the therapeutic mainstay, newer evidence suggests that local excision with 2–3 cm borders of all involved tissue carries a similar prognosis. Local recurrence is common and can be treated with laser ablation. 5 year survival rates are high, and, because of the late age of onset of disease, patients usually die of some illness other than Paget's disease. If an underlying adenocarcinoma is identified, the patients should undergo radical excision and inguinal lymphadenectomy. The prognosis in patients with lymph node involvement is poor.[12]

UNUSUAL VARIETIES OF VULVAR MALIGNANCY

Unusual varieties of vulvar malignancies comprise only 1–2% various types of sarcomas are unusual. Most common sarcomas are leiomyosarcoma and fibrosarcoma. Clinically these tumors appear as small subcutaneous modules, have smooth surfaces, at first freely mobile, later they become fixed to underlying structures.

Vulvar Sarcomas

Sarcomas represent 1–2% of vulvar malignancies and comprise a heterogeneous group of tumors. Leiomyosarcomas are the most common type, representing 33%. Other histological types include fibrosarcomas, neurofibrosarcomas, liposarcomas, rhabdomyosarcomas, angiosarcomas, epithelioid sarcomas and malignant schwannomas.

Treatment

Primary treatment is a wide surgical excision with or without groin dissection. Adjuvant radiation may be helpful for high grade tumors and locally recurrent low grade lesions. Overall survival rate is usually 70%. No recurrence was found in the series from John Hopkins University.

Lymphomas

The genital tract may be involved with primary malignant lymphomas, but more commonly it is a manifestation of systematic disease. In the lower genital tract, the cervix is the most commonly involved, followed by the vulva and the vagina. Most patients are in their third to sixth decade of life. Three-fourths of the cases involve diffuse large cell or histiocytic non-Hodgkin lymphomas and the remainder are nodular or Burkitt lymphomas. Treatment is with surgical excision followed by chemotherapy, and/or radiation, and the overall survival rate is 70%.

Endodermal Sinus Tumor

Malignant germ cell tumors at an extragonadal site presumably arise from the arrested or aberrant migration of primordial germ cells from the embryonic yolk sac endoderm to the genital ridges. Most vulvar cell tumors are endodermal sinus tumors, and there have been 11 cases reported.[13] Most patients are young adults with a median age of 24 years, unlike vaginal yolk sac tumors, which usually occur in infants. Unlike their ovarian counterpart, they are not always associated with elevated serum alpha fetoprotein levels.[13,14] Using cisplatin-based chemotherapy protocols during the past two decades, all reported patients have been cured, regardless of the type of surgery performed, which ranged from radical local excision to radical vulvectomy and lymph node dissection.

METASTATIC TUMORS OF THE VULVA

Most metastatic tumors of the vulva involve the labia majora and the Bartholin's glands. Metastatic tumors account for 8% of all vulvar tumors and in 50% of the cases, the primary tumor arises in the lower genital tract, including the cervix, vagina, endometrium and ovary. In approximately 10% of the cases, the primary site of the metastatic tumor cannot be identified.

REFERENCES

1. Ragnarsson-Olding BK, Nilsson BR, Kanter-Lewensohn LR, et al. Malignant melanoma of the vulva in a nationwide, 25-year study of 219 Swedish females: predictors of survival. Cancer. 1999;86:1285-93.
2. Moxley KM, Fader AN, Rose PG, et al. Malignant melanoma of the vulva: An extension of cutaneous melanoma? Gynecol Oncol. 2011;122:612-7.
3. Aitken DR, Clausen K, Klein JP, et al. The extent of primary melanoma excision. A re-evaluation-how wide is wide? Am Surg. 1983;198:634-41.
4. Day CL Jr, Mihm MC Jr, Sober AJ, et al. Narrower margins for clinical stage I malignant melanoma. N Engl J Med. 1982;306:479-82.
5. Janco JM, Markovic SN, Weaver AL, et al. Vulvar and vaginal melanoma: Case erices and review of current management options including neoadjuvant chemotherapy. Gynecol Oncol. 2013;129:533-7.
6. Podratz KC, Gaffey TA, Symmonds RE, et al. Melanoma of the vulva: an update: Gynecol Oncol. 1983;16:153-68.
7. Kirkwood JM, Strawderman MH, Ernstoff MS, et al. Interferon alfa-2b adjuvant therapy of high-risk resected cutaneous melanoma: The Eastern Cooperative Oncology Group Trial EST 1684. J Clin Oncol. 1996:14:7-17.
8. Chung AF, Woodruff JM, Lewis JL Jr. Malignant of the vulva: a report of 44 cases. Obstet Gynecol. 1975;45:638-46.
9. Copeland LJ, Sneige N, Gershenson DM, et al. Bartholin gland carcinoma. Obstet Gynecol. 1986;67:794-801.
10. Rosenberg P, Simonsen, Risberg B. Adenoid cystic carcinoma of Bartholon's gland: a report of five new cases treated with surgery and radiotherapy. Gynecol Oncol. 1989:34:145-7.
11. Copeland LJ, Sneige N, Gershenson DM, et al. Adenoid cystic carcinoma of Bartholin gland. Obstet Gynecol. 1986;67:115-20.
12. Fortner KB, Szyanki LM, Fox HE, et al. The Johns Hopkins Manual of Gynecology and Obstetrics. Philadelphia: Lippincott Williams and Wilkins; 2010.
13. Kurucu N, Kosucu P, Imamoglu M, et al. Primary vulva endodermal sinus tumor: a case report and review of the literature. Pediatr Int. 2011;53:396-9.
14. Khunamornpong S, Siriaunkgul S, Suprasert P, et al. Yolk sac tumor of the vulva: a case report with long-term disease-free survival. Gynecol Oncol. 2005;97:238-42.

Index

Page numbers followed by *f* refer to figure, and *t* refer to table

A

Acetic acid 50
Adenocarcinoma 65, 110, 113, 114
Adenoid cystic
   carcinomas 110, 112
   tumors 112
Alcock's canal 11
Alcohol injections 26
Aldara 56
American Joint Committee on Cancer Staging for Cutaneous Melanoma 108*t*
Anemia 38
Angiosarcomas 116
Anus 88
Aphthous ulcers 37, 38*f*
Apocrine glands 4
Atopic dermatitis 27
Atopic eczema 27

B

Bartholin's gland 1, 15, 70, 74, 110, 111, 114, 116
   adenocarcinoma of 65
   bilateral 110
   carcinoma 65, 110, 111
      diagnoses of 111
      treatment of 112
   cysts 111
   primary carcinoma of 110, 111
   tumor 111
Basal cell
   carcinoma 65, 112, 113
   hydropic degeneration of 22
Basement membrane, penetration of 49*f*
Behcet's disease 36
Behcet's syndrome 36, 36*f*
Blood sugar-fasting 23
Bowen's cells 43
Bowen's disease 43
Bulbocavernosus body 16
Burkitt lymphomas 116

C

Camper's fascia 83, 84
Cancer, epidermoid 64
Candida albicans 38
Candida infection 28
Carcinoma, adenosquamous 110, 114
Cells, acantholytic 38
Cellular disorganization 40, 48
Cellulites 93
Cervical intraepithelial neoplasia 40
Cervix 117
   colposcopy of 77
Chemoradiation
   primary 112
   therapy 95
Chemotherapy 97
   cisplatin-based 98
   neoadjuvant 97, 112
Clitoral phimosis 21*f*
Clitoris 1, 10-12, 35*f*, 68*f*, 74, 88, 105
   arteries of 12
   lymphatic 13
      drainage of 6*f*, 7*f*
   nerves of 13
   veins of 12
Cloquet's node 74, 83, 85
Crohn's disease 34, 35*f*, 39

D

Darier disease 37
Deep tumor invasion 94
Deep venous thrombosis 93
Diabetes mellitus 38
Dyspareunia 93
Dystrophy, hyperplastic 27
Dysuria 47

E

En block radical vulvectomy 89
Endodermal sinus tumor 65, 116
Endometrium 117
Epidermal growth factor receptor 99
Exophytic cauliflower-like lesion 67
Exophytic growth over
    clitoris 67f
    vulva 67f
External genitalia, nerve supply of 8, 10t
Extracellular matrix protein 19
Eye, inflammatory vacuities of 36

F

Female external genitalia 1, 3f
Fibrosarcoma 115
Fossa ovalis 84f, 85
Foul smell discharge 69f
Fox-Fordyce disease 4, 34, 35f

G

Genital tract epithelium, lower 40
Genitofemoral nerve 8
Glandular structures 1
Glans clitoridis 11
Glans penis 12
Granuloma inguinale 66
Greater vestibular gland 16, 110
Groin
    dissection 83, 89
    lymph nodes, management of 82, 90, 109
    node dissection, ipsilateral 85

H

Hailey-Hailey disease 37
Hair
    bearing skin 2
    follicles 4
        absence of 9
Hemorrhages 93
Hernia, femoral 93
Human papillomavirus 41, 65
    infection 28, 43, 49
    vaccination 57
    vaccine 51
Hydrochloride 26
Hymenal ring 10
Hyperkeratosis 22, 28, 39
Hyperplasia, squamous 27
Hyperplasic dystrophy 19
Hyperplastic epithelial changes, causes of 29
Hypertension 66
Hypogastric artery 12

I

Iliac artery, internal 12
Imiquimod 56
Immature cells, presence of 40
Inflammatory
    cell infiltration, chronic 28
    epithelial disorders 18
    skin, chronic 19
Inguinal canal 4
Inguinal fold 20
Inguinal lymph node 84f
Inguinofemoral node dissection, bilateral 85
International Federation of Gynecology and Obstetrics 72, 73t, 100t, 107
International Society for Study of Vulvar Disease 18
    classification 46
    terminology 42
Intraepithelial neoplasia 46
Introital stenosis 93

Index

K

Keratinocytes, epithelial 56
Keratosis follicularis 37
Koebner response 19
Kraurosis vulvae 43

L

Labia majora 1, 2, 9, 10, 20, 35f, 68f, 70, 116
   arteries of 4f, 5
   deep structures of 3
   lymphatics of 5
   veins of 5
Labia minora 1, 2, 9, 10, 12, 13, 20, 30, 35f, 105
   agglutination of 21f
   arteries of 11
   veins of 11
Labial skin, inner surface of 3
Laser ablation 54
Laser therapy
   advantages of 55
   disadvantages of 55
Leiomyosarcoma 115
Leukoplakia 27, 43, 68f, 71
Lichen planus 19, 27, 30, 31f
Lichen sclerosus 19, 20, 21f, 22, 23, 26, 27, 66
   microscopic feature of 22f
Lichen simplex 23
   chronicus 19, 27
Liposarcomas 115
Liver 39
Local steroid therapy 24
Lupus erythematosus 23
Lymph node 8f, 39, 108
   contralateral 75
   metastases 72, 101
      incidence of 74t
Lymphadenectomy, inguinofemoral 83
Lymphatic
   drainage 14
   mapping 85, 86f
   metastases 72
Lymphocytes, large 93
Lymphogranuloma venereum 66
Lymphoma 65, 116
Lymphovascular space invasion 94

M

Malignant germ cell tumors 116
Malignant lymphomas, primary 116
Melanoma
   benign 106f
   malignant 65, 106f
   superficial spreading 106
Mering procedure 26
Mesonephric ducts 16
Metastatic lymph nodes, number of 108
Metastatic tumor 65, 116
Micrometastatic disease 108
Mons pubis 1, 2, 10
Mucosa, erythematous 30
Mucosal lentiginous melanoma 106
Multifocal disease 54
Multiple condyloma 47
Muscles, ischiocavernosus 12
Myocardial infarction 93

N

National Cancer Institute's Surveillance Epidemiology and End Results Program 42
Nerve 11
Neurodermatitis 27
Neurofibrosarcomas 115
Nodal metastasis 75
Nodular melanoma 106
Non-neoplastic
   epithelial disorders 46
   inflammatory disease 33
Non-pigmented lesions 105
Nonsteroidal anti-inflammatory drugs 52

O

Osteitis pubis 93
Ovary 117

P

Paget's cells 60f, 114
Paget's disease 58, 59f, 61, 62, 65, 110, 113-115
   extramammary 65
   histology of 60f
   invasive 61
   labium majora 60f
   microscopic appearance of 115f
   vulva 110, 114f
      classification of 58
      secondary 58
Pain 15
Papanicolaou smear 70
Parakeratosis 114
Paraurethral ducts 16
Pelvic
   exenteration 91
   lymph nodes, management of 90
Pemphigus
   familial benign chronic 37
   vulgaris 37
Penis 12
Perianal skin 20
Pigmented moles 113
Post-simple vulvectomy 82f
   drain tube in situ 81f
Prepuce 35f
Pruritic papules 35f
Pruritus 47
Psoriasis 19, 27
   sites of 34
Pubic
   osteomyelitis 93
   ramus 112
   symphysis 12

R

Radiation fibrosis 23
Radiation therapy 87, 99, 102
   acute complications of 96
   late complication of 97
   role of 94
   technique 96
Radical local excision 80
Radical vulvectomy 88, 89
Radiotherapy, intensity-modulated 99
Retinoid therapy 25
Rhabdomyosarcomas 116
Rodent ulcer 113

S

Saphenous vein, long 5f
Sarcomas 65
   epithelioid 116
Scleroderma, advanced 23
Seborrheic dermatosis 27
Sentinel lymph node 72, 86
   biopsy 108, 109
Sexually transmitted diseases 66
Simple pruritic maculopapular eruption 113
Skene ducts 16
Skene gland cyst 16
Skinning vulvectomy 54
   indications of 54
Squamous cell
   carcinoma 64, 97
      invasive 41
      of vulva, types of 67
   hyperplasia 19, 27-29, 65, 66
   type 64
Squamous vulvar
   cancer, clinical profile of 69
   intraepithelial neoplasia 42, 43, 45
Sudoriferous glands 4
Superficial epithelium, atrophy of 22
Superficial fascia 84f, 85
Superficial inguinal nodes 14
Sweat glands 3
Swelling 47
Syphilis 66
Systemic disease
   acute phases of 39f
   chronic phases of 39f

T

Testosterone 25
Thyroid
   diseases, autoimmune 19
   stimulating hormone, serum 23

Index

Thyroxine 23
Transitional cell carcinoma 110
Triamcinolone acetonide
 suspension 25
Tumor
 location of 101
 microinvasive 79
 primary 88, 108
 size of 94, 100
 thickness 107

U

Ulcer 37
 herpetic 71
 syphilitic 71
 tubercular 71
Ulcerative vulvar disease 33
Urethra 64, 88, 105
 female 16
Urethral diverticula 17
Urinary tract infection 93

V

Vagina 10, 64, 88, 105, 117
Vaginal adhesions 26
Vaginal introitus 22*f*
Verrucous carcinoma 64, 101
 treatment of 102
Verrucous type lesion 67
Vestibular gland 1, 34
Vestibule 13
 arteries of 14
 lymphatics of 14
 nerves of 14
 veins of 14
Vulva 1, 4*f*, 8*f*, 38*f*
 adenocarcinoma of 114
 colposcopy of 78
 composition of 64
 different parts of 1*f*
 disorder of 33
 hair bearing areas of 59*f*
 lichen planus of 30
 malignant melanoma of 105, 107
 metastatic tumors of 116

mucosa of 46
 primary malignant neoplasms of
  105
 skin of 18
 squamous carcinoma of 68*f*, 70
 squamous cell cancer of 98
 surface anatomy of 7*f*
 tumors of 71
 vestibule of 33
 weeping lesion of 59*f*
Vulvar adenocarcinomas 113
Vulvar adhesions 26
Vulvar cancer 64, 66, 94, 97
 classification of 64
 early diagnosis of 66
 early stage 76
 FIGO staging system for 72
 nonsquamous type of 105
 recurrent 98
 squamous 70, 98
 staging of 78
 surgical staging for 73*t*
 treatment of 78
Vulvar carcinoma 77, 97
 in situ 43
Vulvar denervation 26
Vulvar diffuse white lesions 71
Vulvar diseases 4
Vulvar dystrophy 18, 41, 65, 66, 71
 types of 18
Vulvar eczema 27
Vulvar epithelium 2
Vulvar groin dissection 89
Vulvar intraepithelial neoplasia 40, 41,
  46, 47, 48*f*, 65
 classification of 43
 hyperpigmented 48*f*
 natural history of 44
Vulvar irritation 47
Vulvar lymphatic flow 7*f*
Vulvar malignant melanoma 105
 management of 109
Vulvar melanomas 107
Vulvar preinvasive lesions, high-grade
  50
Vulvar psoriasis 34
Vulvar sarcomas 115

Vulvar skin 20, 40, 75
Vulvar squamous
    cell carcinoma 105
    intraepithelial
        lesion, microscopic appearance
           of 49*f*
        neoplasia, clinical profile
           of 46
Vulvar tumor, primary 94
Vulvar ulcerative lesions 71
Vulvar veins, drainage of 5*f*

Vulvar vestibulitis 33
    syndrome 33*f*
Vulvectomy, simple 54, 80*f*, 81*f*

W

White lesion 47
Wolffian ducts 16
Wound
    closer of 82*f*
    primary closer of 82*f*

EU GSPR Authorised Reprsentative
Logos Europe, 9 rue Nicolas Poussin
1700, La Rochelle, France
Phone: +33 (0) 6 67 93 73 78
E-mail: contact@logoseurope.eu

www.ingramcontent.com/pod-product-compliance
Ingram Content Group UK Ltd.
Pitfield, Milton Keynes, MK11 3LW, UK
UKHW021827140426
5217IPUK00016B/1244